Praise for CAL OREY's
Classic Health Books

The Healing Powers of Superfoods
"Ancient healing wisdom meets modern-day foods in this super book."
—Ann Louise Gittleman, Ph.D., C.N.S.,
author of *The Fat Flush Plan*

"In *The Healing Powers of Superfoods*, we're thankfully
rediscovering these amazingly healthy foods again today."
—Will Clower, Ph.D., CEO, Mediterranean Wellness

The Healing Powers of Tea
"Confirmed enthusiasts of the drink will most appreciate Orey's
well-constructed and comprehensive guide; foodies and those
with an interest in alternative-health therapies will also want
to thumb through it."
—*Publishers Weekly*

"Tea is an ancient elixir that is making quite a therapeutic
comeback. I know this book will be your cup of tea!"
—Ann Louise Gittleman, Ph.D., C.N.S.,
author of *The Fat Flush Plan*

"*The Healing Powers of Tea*, like the drink itself, is a
nourishing comfort."
—Will Clower, Ph.D., CEO, Mediterranean Wellness

The Healing Powers of Vinegar, *Revised and Updated*
"A practical, health-oriented book that everyone who wants to stay
healthy and live longer should read."
—Patricia Bragg, N.D., Ph.D., author of *Apple Cider Vinegar*

"For heart, mind, and body, Cal Orey shows us why coffee is the most comforting health food on the planet."
—Dr. Will Clower, Ph.D., CEO, Mediterranean Wellness

The Healing Powers of Honey
"A fascinating read about a natural remedy that is a rich source of antioxidants."
—Ray Sahelian, M.D., author of *Mind Boosters*

"Not everyone can be a beekeeper, but Cal Orey shares the secrets that honeybees and their keepers have always known. Honey is good for body and soul."
—Kim Flottum, editor of *Bee Culture* magazine and author of several honeybee books

The Healing Powers of Chocolate
"The right kind, the right amount of chocolate may just save your life."
—Ann Louise Gittleman, Ph.D., C.N.S., author of *The Fat Flush Plan*

"Chocolate is a taste of divine ecstasy on Earth. It is our sensual communion. Orey's journalistic style and efforts share this insight with readers around the world."
—Jim Walsh, founder, Intentional Chocolate

Books by CAL OREY

The Healing Powers of Essential Oils

The Healing Powers of Superfoods

The Healing Powers of Tea

The Healing Powers of Coffee

The Healing Powers of Honey

The Healing Powers of Chocolate

The Healing Powers of Olive Oil

The Healing Powers of Vinegar

Doctors' Orders

202 Pets' Peeves

Published by Kensington Publishing Corp.

The
Healing Powers of
Essential Oils

A COMPLETE GUIDE TO NATURE'S MOST MAGICAL MEDICINE

Cal Orey

CITADEL PRESS
Kensington Publishing Corp.
www.kensingtonbooks.com

CITADEL PRESS BOOKS are published by

Kensington Publishing Corp.
119 West 40th Street
New York, NY 10018

All Kensington titles, imprints, and distributed lines are available at special quantity discounts for bulk purchases for sales promotions, premiums, fund-raising, educational, or institutional use. Special book excerpts or cus-tomized printings can also be created to fit specific needs. For details, write or phone the office of the Kensington sales manager: Kensington Publishing Corp., 119 West 40th Street, New York, NY 10018, attn: Sales Department; phone 1-800-221-2647.

ISBN-13: 978-0-8065-3917-1
ISBN-10: 0-8065-3917-8

First trade paperback printing: January 2020

10 9 8 7 6 5 4 3

Printed in the United States of America

Electronic edition: January 2020

ISBN-13: 978-0-8065-3918-8 (e-book)
ISBN-10: 0-8065-3918-6 (e-book)

A special dedication to Mother Nature, my muse behind plant therapy. Healing oils and scents deliver fond memories for all seasons to feel at home wherever I am.

CONTENTS

Foreword

SEA OF SCENTS

It's weird. Sailing on the ocean connects me to something almost primal that pulls at my heart like a love, or maybe an ache. It's hard to describe, but even when I'm close to the ocean and catch the scent of the salty sea, it triggers that thing, that feeling, that essence like inhaling an essential oil smell.

Where does that feeling happen, when you catch an aroma and immediately get whooshed along to an emotional place you never expected? These are the kinds of ridiculous questions my mind dreams up, but I can give you the short answer now. The deep brain.

Along with sailing, I've had so many blessings in my life and none more so than being a neuroscientist. I got to listen to brain cells orchestrate active behavior right in front of me—the animal reaches for the raisin, the brain cell fires; the animal stops, the brain cell stops. It's like being granted access to glimpse the greatest mystery on Earth. If you don't feel a reverence when this happens, you're not paying attention.

One key thing I understood as a neuroscientist is how very little we really know about the brain. This is especially true when I think about the impact aromas have on the mind. That said, at least the clues to unlocking mysteries are there.

For example, the cells on the top layer of the brain fire when you reach for a cup, remember a to-do list, feel the breeze on your skin, or futz with a crossword puzzle. But this conscious portion of your brain is only a small piece of the whole.

But move down deeper, beneath the cortical cares of consciousness, into the lower layers. There you'll find the makings of memories. Feelings and fragments. Sounds and smells that trigger the remnants of joys and disasters you didn't even remember you had forgotten. Their threads still run through this place, where the light of consciousness is dimmer and the musty sensations are far more potent.

This is where the salty sea smells move my soul.

WELCOME TO THE OLFACTORY SENSE OF SMELL

It's no surprise then that the olfactory sense of smell enters these same deep brain structures of the nervous system. In fact, smells entering the olfactory system at the nose have been shown to impact deep brain regions such as the hippocampus and the limbic system. These areas process the signal, then trigger those latent memories and emotions.

Once these subterranean regions get these signals, they can nudge your sense of self in a way that doesn't come from logic or reason above. Think about "new puppy smell," "fresh-baked bread," or "Christmas tree." These all produce reactions inside of us, welling up unconsciously to create a range of emotions.

This effect of certain aromas on behavior is well known. In fact, the action of essential oils on behavior has been known and utilized by medicine for centuries. Unfortunately, over time this understanding receded into a distant medical memory.

A WHIFF OF REVIVAL FOR HEALING OILS

The good news is that there's now a whiff of revival in this more ancient approach. Research has circled back on essential oils, reassessing their properties like a long-forgotten feedback loop that ties together the older practice with our modern scientific understanding.

We are starting to remember what we have forgotten.

Experimental studies have recently shown how essential oils can reduce objective measures of anxiety and stress. These neurobehavioral results are confirmed for cancer patients as well. As you might expect, the outcome seems to be an improved sense of calm—both emotionally and physically.

For women receiving chemotherapy for breast cancer, ginger essential oil lessens acute nausea. For those receiving breast biopsies, exposure to lavender-sandalwood oil reduces measures of anxiety. And for cancer patients having needles inserted, lavender essential oil left them with less pain, as compared to controls who had no such exposure.

Given the connection of the olfactory system to the deep brain structures, these outcomes make perfect sense. And in some ways, these studies confirm what we already knew to be true. This is great news, but even better is the fact that we don't have to wait for all the studies to be done to take advantage of the impact essential oils have on our physical and emotional health.

Cal Orey's latest in the *Healing Powers* series provides a clear and comprehensive look at essential oils: what they are, where they come from, how they are used, how they're used at home, and their health benefits.

The Healing Powers of Essential Oils is also a practical guide that helps incorporate them into your daily life, with over fifty recipes using essential oils. These are not only easy to prepare and delicious to eat, but will fill your home with the wonderful healthful aromas your family will love.

—Will Clower, Ph.D.
CEO, Mediterranean Wellness
Author of *The Fat Fallacy*,
The French Don't Diet, and
Eat Chocolate, Lose Weight

Introduction

So, why did I choose to write a book on essential oils and aromatherapy, anyhow? Let me explain how this *Healing Powers* series number eight bloomed—and take you along on my adventures into the land of Aromatherapy.

Perhaps, my past books were the seeds of a new book budding. After all, olive oil is a healing oil that, like essential oils, goes back to the biblical era, as do honey, chocolate, coffee, and tea. All of these natural wonders come from plants and trees. Essential oils are a spin-off—a different gift from Mother Nature.

I was born and raised in California, so the topic of essential oils and aromatherapy seemed appropriate. After all, I was living amid the sixties and seventies, during the heyday of the magic of oils, scents, and candles. It was a time when patchouli oil and eucalyptus oils were "in" as well as burning sandalwood incense and scented vanilla and lavender candles. It was meant to be for me to write this new book.

All right. I am not a certified aromatherapist or a doctor—but I am a baby boomer who gets the world of healing essential oils. My time served as a health author-journalist who dishes about healing foods to nourish the body, mind, and spirit gave me a ticket into the world of scent. This time around, I have a past of growing up around a hub of plants, trees, and flowers. And throughout the decades I've experienced essential oils from flowers, plants, and trees around the nation, from the West Coast, East Coast, South, Pacific Northwest, and in Canada—all boasting a common link to being the source of a wide variety of essential oils.

So as a nature lover but not a naturopath, plant therapy was nothing new to me. I did connect with essential oil experts from around the nation and world to research this topic. When I wrote a mini mag entitled, *The Magic of Oils, Scents & Candles*, which was published twenty years ago, the first year of the new millennium . . . it was a foreshadowing. I was clueless to how vast the world of aromatherapy and essential oils was, nor did I understand the full magnitude of the medicinal and therapeutic benefits. But now the world of essential oils and aromatherapy is more popular and continues to grow in the twenty-first century.

Go ahead, cozy up and brew a cup of herbal tea, light a scented candle, or spritz your favorite essential oil diluted with water around you. It's time. Turn the pages, one by one, or skip to a section if you choose, but come along with me and enter a world of essential oils that will allow you to discover and escape with me back in time, around the nation and world of oils and scents.

Author's Note

This book is intended as a reference tool only. It does not give medical advice. Be sure to consult your doctor or the appropriate health-care professional before starting any new essential oil or diet.

You'll enjoy Mediterranean Diet–style recipes flavored with a variety of dietary essential oils to provide an extra bit of deliciousness. The essential oil recipes in this book have been tested by me, my family and friends, and/or veteran chefs, bakers, and essential oil commercial companies, and established specialty food organizations. Changing ingredients or using different brands of essential oils may change the results in a recipe.

In some of the chapters, including the topics of home cures, slimming oils, beauty, and household hints, my top 20 essential oils are part of a blend with other healing oils. Take precaution when using essential oils. Some oils should be diluted. Also, I have learned using the savvy toothpick method—dip a toothpick into an essential oil vial—instead of using drops. It is a safer way to monitor how much oil you put into an edible recipe. (Refer to the "Joy of Cooking with Edible Oils" chapter to find out more.)

While flavor to antioxidant and antimicrobial powers comes with essential oils infused in food recipes, less is more. And note, essential oils are more potent than flavoring extracts. So using more will *not* provide better or quicker results.

Do note, references to healing oils are found in the Bible, which I discuss a bit. However, I chose to infuse heartfelt literary quotations in each chapter from famous authors. Their words of wisdom about the plant parts of essential oils, including flowers, leaves, and bark, resonate with me as I hope they do you; without the source there would be no essential oils. The masters give due credit to the plant part that provides us with healing powers of essential oils.

It took a while for me to understand the chemistry makeup of each essential oil. I do share the main compounds in each and every of the 20 oils, and discuss how a lot of these isolated properties do the magic for your body, mind, and spirit. These healing properties are also noted by medical researchers in studies, aromatherapists, and even medical doctors.

Do take note of the glossary at the end of this book. The topic of essential oils can be simple but it also can be full of scientific-ese. Once you get it, like I finally did, you'll discover it's much like pinpointing nutrients in foods and beverages.

Also, you may discover that the world of essential oils contains controversy. Some aromatherapists believe healing oils are kid-friendly and pet-safe. Others disagree. Proponents of essential oils debate about including them in food and beverages. So like other health or nutrition topics, there is controversy in the world of essential oils. My mission is to be objective. I tell it like it is. There is no definitive answer, so I leave conclusions up to you. Come along with me on a fun, intriguing, and informative journey into the world of essential oils. It is a journey that will be adventurous and unforgettable as you learn oil by oil exactly what your nose knows and what essential oils and aromatherapy can do for you.

PART 1

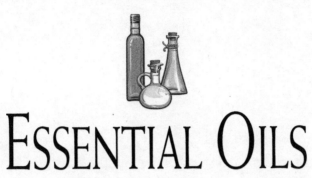

ESSENTIAL OILS

Powerful Healing of Plants

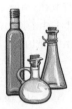

We need the tonic of the wildness.
—HENRY DAVID THOREAU

As a kid, I cherished the dog days of summer in the fragrant purple fields on a small lavender farm in a tiny town in France. Sitting on the porch, sipping lavender-honey lemonade, I scrutinized my dad as he worked hard on our farm with 100,000 lavender plants. One balmy afternoon before dusk I recall he gestured to me to help him. It was my job to hold the gigantic burlap bags open while he, a strong man with weathered skin, dropped bunches of lavender bundles into it. The pungent and pine scent of picturesque lilac flowers in this countryside paradise takes me back in time, back to nature.

I ran back to our house, into the rustic kitchen, and brought a gift to my mom.

"Thank you, dear. Lavender oil for the Bundt cake glaze will be picture-perfect," she exclaimed, touching her big belly with my sibling soon to be born. The extraction method for lavender oil was old school, not like buying a vial of the essential oil. My mom would combine a vegetable oil with dried lavender in a large container and then sun-dry it for weeks before it was ready to use.

She let me sprinkle sprigs of lavender into the yellow batter and fold it in until it was dispersed. The spice cake in the oven filled the warm air with a bit of essential oils, cinnamon, thyme, and lemon aroma. Once baked and cooled, it was my job to drizzle a lavender oil glaze on top of the Bundt cake.

"Impeccable!"

My mother's declaration made me feel good, but I didn't know what the word meant. What I did know, however, was that the aromatic cake was like walking into a French bakery in town, full of fresh scents to love.

Okay. So, this slice of life in Europe is in my imagination. But in real life my mother did bake. She did use lavender from our backyard garden during the summer and infused it with olive oil. I was often her sous chef, as she would say. And while I didn't grow up in a farmhouse surrounded by purple flowers, my mother did go to France one time and I did end up having a younger brother to share my life then and now.

Truthfully, I was raised in a suburb of Northern California; but I have learned because of our Mediterranean climate, prevalent up and down the West Coast, lavender fields and farms did and still do exist in the Golden State. And I am certain there was a mother and a daughter who created lavender baked goods with lavender oil in their kitchen as I imagined we did.

In my youth I really did eat and enjoy home-baked foods infused with essential oils (yes, cake with hints of lavender oil made from scratch). Born and raised in a middle-class suburban lifestyle, I still have images of fresh homegrown backyard herbs and spices mixed with vegetable oil. During the mid-twentieth century, we used homemade oils like this or dried herbs and spices or the herbs and spices in cans. I don't recall seeing dietary essential oils in vials stocked in our kitchen pantry or available to order online since we didn't have computers. We used DIY essential oils. But times changed.

Nowadays, essential oils are convenient to obtain, cost-effective, and used in cooking and baking. After all, lemons, for instance, are not always available year-round, but lemon essential oil can be in your pantry whenever you need it. And that is where essential oils come into the picture because they are there for you anytime, anywhere. As a Golden State health-nut foodie, I can look back at my life growing up, decade by decade, and understand how nature's garden, including homemade to store-bought essential oils, has played a role in my real world.

A TIME FOR ESSENTIAL OILS

While I'm not living on a lavender farm, I can smell the lavender essential oil I use and store in my kitchen and bathroom and that keeps on giving me a healthy balance. In fact, I am currently wearing an aromatherapy necklace and just sniffed the down-to-earth lavender essential oil to help keep calm and centered. In the twenty-first century, we are living in a hectic pace and we often don't stop to smell the lavender (it wouldn't survive in a dry, cold winter), nor take time to pamper ourselves. By infusing aromatherapy (nature's essential oils and candles) and aromachology (mood-changing scents) to your daily regime, perhaps you, like me, can slow down, take a deep breath, exhale, and feel better by nourishing your mind, body, and spirit, effortlessly with the power of aromas!

Stacks of research, past and present, have shown that specific smells, like lavender, affect the limbic or pleasure center of the brain, inducing a sense of well-being and happiness, boosting the hormone serotonin, which makes us feel good, like after exercising or making love, or eating a piece of chocolate. And happy people are more balanced, and may even live longer, healthier lives, thanks to essential oils and aromatherapy.

AROMATHERAPY BASICS 101

So, what exactly is aromatherapy? It's the use of essential oils from aromatic plants to relax, balance, rejuvenate, restore and enhance the body, mind, and spirit. And essential oils, huh? You can stop wondering what they are because I'm here to dish the lowdown on everything you want to know but were too afraid or busy to ask.

Essential oils are extracted from the bark, leaves, petals, resins, rinds, roots, seeds, stalks, and stems of aromatic plants. They're the concentrated part of a plant—the true essence of flowers, fruits, or spices that are believed to have a powerful effect on a person's overall mood and much, much more.

The healing powers of essential oils are no secret. Like me, people use essential oils not only as home cures but also as a weight loss, heart-healthy, and anti-aging prescription, where it provides limitless healing powers.

There is a crazy limitless amount of information to discover and experience firsthand about essential oils.

The Essential Term for Essential Oils

Essential oil: any of a class of volatile oils that give plants their characteristic odors and are used especially in perfumes and flavorings and for aromatherapy.
—Merriam-Webster

Medical doctors and essential oil medical researchers continue to discover new findings about nature's oils, from past and present-day. It's not just about lavender or ginger—two popular herbs and essential oils. People, like you and me, are discovering just what nature's herbalists have been saying for centuries—essential oils do indeed have surprising healing powers.

Valerie Ann Worwood, the author of *The Complete Book of Essential Oils*, points out that essential oils give us an aromatic pharmacy chock-full of remedies and delights for usage in our lives.[1]

Kathie Keville, who wrote *Aromatherapy for Dummies*, also notes, "If the plant has a scent, it contains essential oils," which means flowers, herbs, and even trees that surround you in your environment owe their distinctive aromas to essential oils.[2]

Dr. Ann Louise Gittleman says, "Essential oils are all the rage. Whether you're seeking a specific ailment or simply want a safe scent to fill your home, essential oils provide a wide array of therapeutic benefits." But she knows healing oils are nothing new.

Countless health experts, like Dr. Gittleman, and others in both unconventional and conventional medicine, are coming around to accepting the power of essential oils. Essential oils and aromatherapy are a no-nonsense topic that people around the world have embraced for centuries.

MEET THE FAVORITE ESSENTIAL OILS

Today, we know more about the ancient medicine behind essential oils than ever before. There are hundreds of essential oils from plants, but there seems to be a few dozen that pop up again and again, whether you're talking to seasoned aromatherapists, or just people who like essentials oils, spas, and beauty products. And this usage of nature's pharmacy is not a fad; there is hard-hitting proof that essential oils can and do help you feel and look better, as well as add super quality years to your life.

In fact, essential oils have been called "ancient medicine" due to the fact they can be traced back to the biblical era. And it's no surprise some of these oils are considered essential because a number of them are connected with lowering the development of cancer, diabetes, heart disease, and much more. But how? How can they keep us healthy?

Medical researchers believe antioxidants act like pharmaceuticals (which are currently being researched for their potential to treat diseases and stall aging). You wouldn't think essential oils would contain disease-fighting antioxidants like the top antioxidant-rich foods—but they do! Surprise. Antioxidants are the "super warriors" who, like Pac-Man in the video game, gobble up the enemies that can make you sick. The antioxidant warriors protect our bodies' cells from damaging effects of free radicals, the rivals that can cause health problems.

Essential oils do contain the same antioxidants and can be effective in many different ways—not just consuming edible oils in foods. According to the ORAC (Oxygen Radical Absorbance Capacity)—the amount of antioxidant power in a food (or essential oil)—*many of* my top 20 oils are in the top ranking.

ORAC VALUES OF TOP ESSENTIAL OILS

You may think providing the numbers linked to nature's antioxidants isn't important but think again. This sampling of essential oils and ORAC score ranking shows that healing oils can be rated—and can be used topically, inhaled, or with some, even ingested for their benefits.

Oil	ORAC score (per 100 grams)
Cedarwood	169,000
Clove	1,078,700
Myrrh	379,800
Cedarwood	169,000
Geranium	101,000
Ginger	99,300
Basil	54,000
Patchouli	49,400
Cinnamon	10,340

After studying a variety of antioxidant (ORAC) scores for essential oils, it's puzzling because some numbers don't match. The truth is, the ORAC scale was created by USDA researchers at Tufts University. Also, it's a fact that essential oils like superfoods do indeed have high scores. Other essential oils that have super high ORAC scores include German chamomile, patchouli, peppermint, rose, and sage. There's no need to dole out more numbers. All you need to know is that essential oils are rich in antioxidants and are healthy for you.

It's crucial to add now, you will not be using 100 grams (3 ounces) of an essential oil, whether it's inhaled, used topically, or consumed. It is a very small amount (1 drop to a toothpick bead for cooking and baking) because essential oils are concentrated and therefore four times more potent than a food extract! However, that doesn't mean you will *not* get the good antioxidant disease-fighting benefits. You will. And when you use essential oils diluted with carrier oils like olive oil, jojoba oil, or coconut oil, you are receiving even more healing compounds for your body.

WHAT'S SO ESSENTIAL ABOUT ESSENTIAL OILS?

Essential oils are not just about benefiting from the multiple healing powers of their disease-fighting antioxidants. In medical studies, scientists give credit to specific properties in the oils that are linked to both medicinal and therapeutic healing powers. There are dozens and dozens of compounds; however, certain ones continue to pop up again and again, and it's these superstars that I will introduce to you.

Meet three chemical components: phenylpropanoids, monoterpenes, and sesquiterpenes. It is this almighty trio that provides healing powers to essential oils and may be beneficial in aiding illnesses and diseases.[3]

But if you dig deeper into the chemistry composition of essential oils, like I did, there are more groups of properties in essential oils that are linked to specific healing powers. These healing compound categories include, acids, alcohols, aldehydes, esters, terpenes, ketones, and phenols. And the breakdown of isolated components in these groupings include hundreds of constituents. I focus on the main compounds in my 20 essential oil picks. Certain compounds in specific essential oils have been discovered by scientists, and if you do the research, you'll see the same properties in medical journals.[4] Medical research shows which compounds may be why an essential oil can be helpful because they can do different things, such as fighting bacterial, fungal and viral infections, lessening inflammation, stimulating blood circulation, and brainpower as well as enhancing emotions.

The thing is, despite some conventional medical doctors who don't believe essential oils are noteworthy, stacks of studies—on humans, petri dishes, and rodents—show how the components work and provide healing powers. That means, essential oils have made their mark, past and present, in literature and medical journals. The compounds and the synergistic effect of properties within essential oils are making aromatherapy a growing phenomenon that can help enhance our lives and well-being.

We're going to be talking about the most popular universal oils—favorite ones that are found and used today in home cures, beauty treatments, enhancing the household and work environment, and even in cuisine. It's important to understand these oils are derived from plants growing around the world. Most of my 20 picks have roots in Mediterranean countries but are also grown wild and on farms in the United States and other countries. All of the essential oils in the group can be paired in blends with Mediterranean oils and/or in cuisine from the Mediterranean Diet.

THE ESSENTIAL PLANT PARTS PRODUCTION

Plant gardens and essential oils are connected like a growing romance. *Love Blossoms* is a Hallmark film about a perfume maker on a mission to complete her late dad's last unfinished scent. Fate pairs her up with a botanist tending a garden and he has an uncanny, keen sense of smell. The romantic connection of plants and essential oils, like this man and woman, made sense to me—we wouldn't have one without the other. Here, take a glance at where essential oils come from. Your favorite oil may not come from a flower but a tree!

Most of my 20 top picks of essential oil extractions are steam-distilled from parts of plants. People who understand plant therapy, like Dr. Gittleman, point out essential oils "are the life blood of the plant." I heard this term years ago; I understand it better now. Plants are the lifeline to the essential oils we love and use.

Here is a quick glance at a basic breakdown of the plant and oil connection that you can see in gardens.

Part of Plant	Essential Oils
Bark	Cinnamon
Flowers and leaves	Basil, chamomile, lavender, peppermint, sage, spearmint
Flowers, petals, and buds	Chamomile, jasmine, lavender, orange, rose

Part of Plant	Essential Oils
Leaves	Basil, cinnamon, eucalyptus, geranium, patchouli, peppermint, rosemary, spearmint, tea tree
Peel, rind	Lemon, orange
Roots	Ginger
Woods	Cedarwood, sandalwood

THE SCIENCE OF AROMA AND MOOD

Aromachology is an idea based on scientific studies. It is believed by scientists, like Dr. Will Clower, who shares his passionate words about how the scent of the sea makes him feel. That happiness to relaxation stems from smell and the limbic system known as the "pleasure center" of the brain that controls your memory.

Aromatherapy, on the other hand, focuses on the therapeutic effects of aromas on physical conditions from aches and pains to coughing and a sore throat. Aromachology, though, focuses on the therapeutic results aromas can have on stress, anxiety, mood, and memory.

Luxury health spa resorts use aromacology and aromatherapy. This, in turn, can help to reduce stress, promote calmness, boost mood and balance, and improve quality of life and longevity.

So now that you understand my enthusiasm to share my new findings about essential oils, especially versatile favorites that you can find in health food stores and online, also in many household and beauty products at the grocery store, it's time to cozy up with this essential book. Light a scented candle, take a deep breath or two, and inhale. Your nose knows what scents trigger good feelings for you, and I can tell you how each one can be healing from head to toe. Go ahead—whip up a fruit juice beverage infused with a small drop of citrus essential oil (for the refreshing scent and flavor) to get in the right frame of mind to be open for adventure in discovering oils and aromatherapy that'll help you feel so good and so energized.

Essentially Invigorating Garden-Fresh Smoothie

It's time to enjoy a wake-up morning or afternoon fruit smoothie to sip and savor while you sit down or lie down and digest the following pages, one by one, about essential oils and aromatherapy and how they can help you feel alive! This recipe is down-to-earth, California fruit–inspired, and one of my favorites year-round.

½ cup fresh squeezed oranges
½ cup fresh or frozen berries (blueberries or strawberries)
¾ cup organic low-fat milk
¼ cup plain Greek yogurt
1 teaspoon raw honey
1 drop lemon essential oil
½ teaspoon ground cinnamon
Mint sprigs, fresh (for garnish)

Blend juice fruit, milk, and yogurt. Mix in honey and lemon oil and blend again. Then pour into a glass. Sprinkle with cinnamon and top with mint.

Makes 2 servings.

SCENT-SATIONAL HEALING OILS SHORT & SWEET

Research in the latter part of the twentieth century and early twenty-first century shows that essential oils, which come from nature's plants, have healing powers that

✓ Bolster the immune system, naturally.
✓ Reduce the odds of developing cancer.

✓ Enhance Zen-like rest, relaxation, and better sleep.
✓ Boost mood, lessen anxiety and stress.
✓ Lower risk of heart disease.
✓ Fight inflammation and infection.
✓ Aid mindfulness, focus, and memory.
✓ Provide physical energy and stamina.
✓ Keep your spirit alive and the planet healthier.

In this book, I will show you how easily essential oils can be nature's ancient magical medicine for you in the present day. But many people, perhaps you, will not want to reap the benefits of *all* essential oils. So, if you don't like one oil, there are substitutes. You can use essential oils and aromatherapy in a variety of useful ways, both medicinal and therapeutic.

But first, let's go way, way back into the past. Come with me. I'm going to take you to different times, to different places—to Mediterranean regions I've never been and places I did experience or aspire to go to in the future—all for the sake of understanding the roots of essential oils and aromatherapy. Let me show you the fascinating history and folklore of essential oils and how nature's medicine made and is making a gigantic splash around the world and in mainstream culture.

History Of Essential Oils

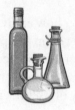

The physician treats, but nature heals.
—HIPPOCRATES

My first real-life essential oils and aromatherapy event happened one Christmas Eve; it is the first one that I recall and will always cherish. As a sensitive kid with a keen sense of smell, the variety of scents on this occasion made a lasting impression on me, like it did characters in the film *Michael*. An archangel played by John Travolta had a distinct scent, a cookie-like aroma that attracted women like a magnet—just like my nose to the array of holiday festivities.

At the end of the day, my dad brought a present into our living room. My eyes feasted on a gigantic fresh pine tree complete with a woodsy aroma. We decorated it with a mix of red, green, and white bulb ornaments. My mom let us hang fresh gingerbread man cookies (ginger oil was used in them) on the branches next to red-and-white-striped candy canes—both the peppermint and ginger scents were strong, like walking into a candy store. It was tradition that after leaving cookies and milk on the dining room table for Santa Claus, my siblings and I would go to bed early. At midnight I was awakened by the sound of "Ho, ho, ho!" and the front door slammed. Running out into the living room, my dad announced it must have been Santa— and now he could build a fire for which he used cedar chips to ignite. My two siblings and my parents sat around the crackling fire, a room full of nature's festive scents. We opened our presents. That year I wanted a Barbie doll, but because they were sold out, Midge (her freckle-faced best friend) was my gift. I was disappointed, but rough-housing with my Dalmatian, Casey, was an everlasting *real* memory— especially due to the ginger oil aroma with other scents, like an essential oil in a gift set, that worked together like instruments in a symphony. In the morning at mass, the priest at Saint Francis Cabrini would swing a thurible, a metal censer attached to chains, full of burn-ing frankincense incense. It was a blessing ritual that I didn't get as a Catholic catechism student, but the scent was calming and he was en-tertaining, like watching a dragon walk past the pews and parishioners.

Every holiday season, like this one, complete with an abundance of oils and aromatherapy, is unforgettable. Each time I smell an essential oil, like ginger, it brings back recollections of Christmas. But this plant therapy goes further back in time than when I was an innocent kid who believed in Santa Claus. Let's take a peek at how essential oils were used during biblical times.

THE GARDEN OF EDEN

In the book of Genesis, Adam and Eve are located in a garden with flowers, trees, and aromatic plants. As a child, in catechism we talked about this nirvana. However, it is believed to be a myth by some reli-gions and academics alike. True or not, the image of God's creation of man and woman amid a beautiful scented parkland is one to cherish.

Despite your beliefs of the garden in the beginning of time, essen-tial oils were indeed appreciated and noted in the Old and New Testaments. Essential oils, their plant sources, and their uses are actu-ally mentioned in the bible a whopping 1,035 times, according to the *Healing Oils of the Bible*'s author, David Stewart.[1]

In the Bible, the two most mentioned oils are frankincense and myrrh, followed by hyssop, spikenard, and wormwood. Next up are balm, cedarwood, myrtle, and aloes. Other oils mentioned are mustard oil, cypress, cinnamon, cumin, juniper, calamus, cassia, dill, coriander, henna, mint, pine, rose, anise, bay leaf, bdellium, rue, saffron, galbanum, and onycha. In my top 20 picks, I include cedarwood, cinnamon, mint, and rose, but you will notice some of these other oils included in blends for home cures and beauty recipes.[2]

Essential oils were used by different peoples of the Bible, such as the Israelites, who often used many oils, including cedarwood, and the early Christians, who weren't strangers to oils like frankincense (what I smelled as a kid at church). Oils were used by different cultures, including the Arabians, Babylonians, Egyptians, and in other regions around the Mediterranean. People used both medicines and perfumes derived from aromas and utilized the healing capabilities from essential oils.[3]

The use of aromatic oils can be traced back forty-five hundred to five thousand years ago in Egypt. The first documented uses of essential oils are from Mesopotamia, China, and India. Back in 3500 B.C. Mesopotamia (aka Southeastern Asia), distillation pots were used and later found at Tepe Gawra. It's believed India used aromatic plants as part of the ayurvedic medical treatments.

Greeks, Romans, and Arabians followed in using essential oils. You may find, as I did, the chronological order of cultures using essential oils in ancient times may differ from sources. Perhaps the different timelines exist because different cultures were using healing oil at the same time. So dates overlap.

An Essential Gift To The Egyptians . . .

In Egypt fragrant herbs were used in aromatherapy for medicinal healing powers and in cosmetics for beauty uses, too. It is also believed Egyptians used a blend of essential oils, which were made from a combination of plants, including resins, barks, and spices. Perhaps the aromatic oils' most popular use was as a way to preserve deceased bodies during the burial process. The young Egyptian King Tut was buried in a tomb surrounded by dozens of alabaster jars filled with essential oils. It was believed that these healing oils were to help him in the afterlife.

Cleopatra's Essential Rose Bath

As the legend goes and is told by aromatherapists and historians, Cleopatra, the Egyptian Queen, and rose water have a sweet-scented history. Rose was used as a fragrance in her aromatherapy baths to keep her skin smooth and soft. It is believed that both she and her lover Mark Antony, a ruler of Rome, pampered themselves with roses in a blend with other scents, including neroli (from orange blossoms)—another floral essential oil. We know that rose water can help make your skin feel soft, but nobody knows for sure if Cleopatra and Antony also used aromatic oils for love scents.

... BLOSSOMED TO CHINA, INDIA, GREECE, AND ROME

China to India: It is documented that essential oils' multitude of benefits were acknowledged and even used by powerful people. The consensus is that aromatic healing oils were used in China dating back to 2697 B.C.E. It is believed during the reign of Huang Ti, essential oils derived from healing herbs and plants were treasured in Eastern medicine, and they are still used for healing powers in the twenty-first century.

China was enjoying essential oils and so was India. Scented plants and oils played a role in the Indian Ayurveda healing powers for at least three thousand years.

Greece and Rome: Greece also enjoyed the benefits of nature's healing gift. History shows Greek soldiers used a medicinal oil from myrrh during war to prevent the infection of wounds. Fragrance played a big role in peoples' lives from royalty and peasants to pharaohs and priests. Aromatherapists will tell you priests were known to lead double lives as perfumers and doctors.

Hippocrates, the Greek father of medicine, shared his forward-thinking talents of treating people with plants. Another well-known healing man in Greece, Galen, also utilized plants and their healing powers. Both doctors studied the medicinal classifications and compounds of plants and their work has not stopped. They were the pioneers of the essential oils of yesteryear that are still being studied in present-day.

The Romans also appreciated fragrant essential oils for body and beauty benefits. In Rome, healing oils were used in baths and for therapeutic massages. After the fall of the Roman Empire, the Dark Ages period arrived. During these troubled times, millions of Europeans were affected by the bubonic plague. The blend of infection-fighting antibacterial essential oils was touted to be a protective and preventative formula used to stave off contracting the deadly pandemic.

Four Thieves Essential Oils Miracle Medicine

During the Middle Ages, essential oils made their imprint on saving lives, too. As the popular legend goes, four robbers in the French town of Marseilles went to homes to take belongings left behind by the victims of the Black Death in Europe. The thieves stayed healthy and immune to the lethal contagion while looting plague-ridden possessions due to a blend they wore during their scavenging.

The original creator of the ancient Four Thieves Formula is unknown. Also, recipes vary with ingredients. The recipe, which uses essential oils, can be made from scratch and can be put to work in many ways. Some people use it to wash down surfaces in an infected room or spritz the air. When diluted with various ingredients like vinegar, it can be used to wash away germs as a body wash. Other people have ingested this magical natural concoction as a precaution—like taking a vitamin to bolster the immune system to fight off a cold or flu. (See the recipe at the end of this chapter.)[4]

THE TWENTIETH-CENTURY ESSENTIAL OILS PARADE

At the turn of the century, doctors and dentists, as well as other types of medical practitioners around the globe, used essential oils and aromatherapy. This trend continued to grow and blossom, decade by decade. People branched out, so to speak, and used a garden variety of plant therapy from essential oils—not just the most popular oils such as lavender and chamomile. Actually, there are reportedly at least three hundred essential oils, according to aromatherapists!

In 1910, as it is noted by numerous historians, a French cosmetic chemist named Rene-Maurice Gattefosse badly burned his hand in a laboratory accident. He put his hand in the nearest liquid—lavender oil—and to his amazement, he discovered that the plant oil led to relief of pain and quick healing. As time passed, Gattefosse studied the medicinal benefits of other plant oils. In fact, in 1937, he published his work and the word "aromatherapy" was coined.

During the twentieth century, another French forward-thinking essential oils enthusiast, Jean Valet, a doctor, started using oils to treat medical ailments including diabetes. He was a pioneer in the world of essential oils as part of treatments for doctors who use them in their practice or even hospitals

In the 1950s, Marguerite Maury started diluting essential oils in carrier oils for massage purposes. Also, she is noted for combining specific oils for specific health ailments.

I lived through the growth of essential oils during the 1960s hippie era, a time of going back to nature. Some essential oils, including chamomile and patchouli, were household names. Many commercial colognes and perfumes were infused with oils. Not to forget the plethora of other oils from bark, flowers, plants, trees, and seeds that were used for home cures and aromatherapy, too, and some were even homemade like basil oil.

In the beginning of the twenty-first century, I got acquainted with more than a dozen essential oils and the devices to use them, especially for beauty care and the household. Twenty years later, I find myself experiencing a wider world of aromatherapy and essential oils, and the therapeutic uses are infinite! And now I know. I know that essential oils are so much more than just something to put on your wrist or in a massage. These days healing oils are a part of my health regimen. I utilize them to help lower the risk of developing age-related diseases, to enhance my mood, and also for cleaning, cooking and baking, and yes, beauty care, too.

PAST MEDICAL USES OF ESSENTIAL OILS

The highlights below are gleaned from a consensus of aromatherapists and historians—I refrain to give credit to one individual source since they do not have definitive proof of these events. Here, take a look at who may be behind essential oils, what feats they likely accomplished, and how they put these wonders to work.

Historical User	Method/Action	Uses
Shen Nung	Wrote book on botanicals	The *Herbal Book* provided medical uses
Queen Hatsheput, Ruler of Egypt	Traveled to Punt and brought back myrrh trees	Used for medicinal purposes
Alexander the Great	Burned incense	Used for health benefits
Cleopatra, Queen of Egypt	Opened an aromatic shop, penned a book named *Cleopatra Gynaeciarum Libri*	Recipes with essential oil combinations used for beauty products, cosmetics, and perfumed ointments.
Pliny, a Roman scholar	Wrote *Natural History* book	Educates people about essential oils
Avicenna, physician	Made essential oils from flowers	Used for healing powers
Dr. Jean-Claude	Conducts research on performing distillation of essential oils	To improve health

OTHER ESSENTIAL MILESTONES

So, during my research for this book, I went to work and learned from herbalists and aromatherapists, and historians. Century by century, I discovered which essential oils were most popular. It's interesting to see how nature's plants were used in the earlier centuries before my time. What is not surprising is that the past repeats itself, or maybe these natural remedies just never faded from our shared human memory at all.

980–1087 A.D.: Ali-Ibn of Persia is behind the discovery of distilling essential oils. The young doctor wrote about hundreds of plants.

1300s: German Saint Hildegard of Bingen made her mark in medicine with plant therapy. Her Physica, a large chronicle of plants and their medicinal effects was published.

1500s: During the time of the bubonic plague in Europe, survivors burned Frankincense and lavender in the streets to prevent the contagion from spreading.

1700s: *The Complete Herbal* was written by an English botanist. The tome was a guide on herbal cures and is still noted in the twenty-first century.

1800s: European researchers studied health benefits of essential oils and their compounds.

PLANT THERAPY MILESTONES IN THE TWENTIETH AND TWENTY-FIRST CENTURIES

Here are a few highpoints of different times the healing powers of essential oils made a splash in the mainstream media, everyday peoples' lives, and my time growing up in the last half of the 1900s.

Year	What Happened	What It Did
1940s	Dr. Jean Valet used essential oils for patients	Helped validate healing powers for injured soldiers
1950s	Austrian Marguerite Maury diluted essential oils in carrier oils, massaging it into skin	The healing of essential oils with vegetable oils became an accepted therapeutic method
1970s	Companies promote essential oils	Plant therapy movement
2000s	Essential oils are infused in beauty care	Consumer demand soared for essential oil—infused products at spas worldwide
2000s	Essential oils are added to household cleaning products, such as dish soap	Aromatic, natural cleaners accepted in the mainstream
2000s	Aromatherapy, including candles, incense, sprays, and diffusers	Aromatherapy usage expands at hotels, spas, medical offices, households
2000s	Aromatherapy uses essential oils for health ailments and diseases	Aromatherapists and holistic doctors include essential oils in their work and for their patients

As you can see, essential oils have been widely recognized for their remarkable medicinal qualities, both in ancient times and today. Essential oils are crazy versatile. Some may believe they can just be used for perfume, much like olive oil is sometimes believed to be only used in a salad dressing. Both ancient healing oils contain medicinal compounds that make them useful in treating the whole body. Speaking of olive oil . . .

MEASURING OILS, DILUTING DROPS

It's important as we visit the top 20 essential oils that you know the basics for your health's sake. A friend of mine, a busy millennial mom, was excited when I told her I was going to gift her with a variety of essential oils for her birthday. I had qualms when she said, "How do you use them?" I was haunted by images of her two children and beloved dog getting into these vials full of essential oils that are so much more potent than the vanilla extract she uses to make cookies. My exaggerated worst-case nightmare would be essential oil overdosing her family. For days I delayed giving the gift of a variety of oils with specific uses, methods, and some cautions.

Before *you* dive into the new world of essential oils, like my pal, it's good to know that when using essential oils, more times than not, they need to be diluted with liquids and/or carrier oils. Yes, they might be ancient medicine from nature's pharmacy, but that doesn't mean they're always safe to use. Do a skin patch test first. Put one diluted drop on your skin. Wait for twenty-four hours. A common dilution is six to twelve drops of essential oil to an ounce of carrier oil, but the ratio of combining a carrier oil with an essential oil varies depending on the recipe. If you see any redness, or other negative effects, do not use.

Consult with your doctor before using essential oils if you're pregnant, have high blood pressure, epilepsy, open wounds, diabetes, rashes, neurological disorders, or if you're taking a prescription medication or homeopathic remedies. Do not swallow essential oils unless they are food-grade quality. For baths or air diffusion, dilute essential oils in water.

And note, dilution measurements of healing oils can differ for many reasons, such as thickness of oil and measurement tools. There are measurement conversion calculators you can use online. Here is a basic essential oils dilution guide for your convenience.

CARRIER	1% ESSENTIAL OIL	2% ESSENTIAL OIL
5 ML	1 DROP	2 DROPS
10 ML	2 DROPS	4 DROPS
0.5 OZ.	3 DROPS	8 DROPS
1 OZ.	6 DROPS	12 DROPS
2 OZ.	12 DROPS	0.25 TSP.
4 OZ.	0.25 TSP.	0.5 TSP.
6 OZ.	36 DROPS	0.75 TSP.
8 OZ.	0.5 TSP.	1 TSP.
16 OZ.	1 TSP.	2 TSP.

(Courtesy of Mountain Rose Herbs.)

Multipurpose Carrier Oils: To use essential oils, both internally and externally, you'll need to use carrier oils, which are oils that can be used to dilute pure essential oils. Simply put, carrier oils are extracted from different sources, such as kernels, nuts, seeds, and other parts of healing plants—and often essential to dilute with essential oils. Carrier oils aid in diluting potent essential oils and they help conserve the use of costly essential oils such as rose oil.

After you get to know the top 20 essential oils and home cures, you will have a better handle on what specific carrier oils work with each essential oil—and which ones work best for you. But for now, here is a quick guide for you to follow:

Almond oil: used for body oils, massage, and perfumes.

Coconut oil: used for healing and lubricating skin; cooking and baking.

Jojoba oil: used for body oils, facial oils, massaging and soothing skin, and perfumes.

Olive oil: a light oil, used for healing and nourishing skin; extra virgin olive oil is best for cooking and baking.

Sesame oil: used for massage, and cooking.

As for my young friend who was enthusiastic to try essential oils? I ended up giving her an aromatherapy diffuser necklace. You simply put a few drops of an undiluted essential oil on a small pad and insert it into a locket on its chain. No carrier oil needed. Also, I asked her to promise me that she would store the essential oils in a safe, dark place—away from children and pets. She was thrilled by the scents of energizing peppermint and the subtle aroma of lavender . . . and I was calm knowing I did my part for a newbie, like I used to be.

In other parts of this book, I'll expound on more safety tips regarding specific essential oils since not one bottle fits all. Some chapters at the end and the recipes chapter do include recipes with food-grade essential oils. Again, refer to chapter 29 to discover more specific directions about cooking and baking with essential oils before consuming oils so you can do so with peace of mind—like I did!

Infection-Fighting
Four Thieves Formula

In the top 20 essential oils highlighted in this book, I include these oils, excluding rue oil and plantain oil. This formula is popular and still gains attention when there is a flu or superbug outbreak and antibiotics do not work.

3 quarts apple cider vinegar
1 drop basil oil
1 drop rosemary oil
1 drop lavender oil
1 drop sage oil
1 drop mint oil
1 drop rue oil
1 drop plantain oil
6 cloves garlic

Combine vinegar with essential oils and garlic. Let the mixture sit in a covered container for at least 24 hours. This may be used on surfaces in a room, topically on the body, and 1 or 2 drops can be consumed sparingly. As with carrier oils, since it is diluted with vinegar (also a carrier), you are getting less rather than more.

In the next chapter, you'll be entering the incredible world of healing essential oils as I take you into the twentieth and twenty-first centuries, a time when plant therapy was and still is a phenomenon. These days, people use essential oils and aromatherapy solo or in a blend for a synergistic effect—and either way can be life changing for the mind and body.

SCENT-SATIONAL HEALING OILS SHORT & SWEET

✓ Remember, essential oils can be traced back to ancient times, when nature's pharmacy was used for major medicinal purposes and minor health ailments.

✓ Aromatherapy and essential oils were publicized for their healing powers, by the Egyptians, Greeks, Romans, and other peoples who put to use the natural multipurpose virtues of plant therapy.

✓ By the fifteenth century, essential oils were used in London by especially royalty (but peasants, too) who infused healthful food with healing oils as well as used them for medical benefits.

✓ In the eighteenth century, medical researchers in Europe studied components in essential oils. Healing oils were used and prescribed by pharmacies.

✓ Caution: Use common sense when you hear claims of miracle essential oil health cures. Consider advantages and disadvantages of specific oils. (Refer to the end of each of the 20 essential oil chapters before you try a healing method.)

✓ Since scientists do not have proof that one essential oil is a cure-all for one disease, monitor your personal reaction—no oil fits all.

✓ Keep in mind, essential oils are most effective when a variety of them are used—like eating a variety of wholesome foods to benefit from numerous healing compounds.

PART 2

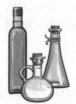

TOP 20 POPULAR
ESSENTIAL OILS

OPENING UP 20 AROMATIC BOTTLES

The top 20 essential oils I've selected in part 2 may make you smile, and you will likely have your special preferences, because they are the darlings of the oils used around the world. It is like having a basic wardrobe of essential oils to build on. And, of course, blending other essential oils and using different methods to glean their healing powers can work wonders for you, too.

While I chose *my* favorite essential oils, and share their botanical names, I was surprised that many of my picks are ones that mainstream America loves, too. Seventy-five percent of the mixed bag of essential oils I chose have strong Mediterranean roots from the past. The other handful of oils, such as cinnamon, ginger, patchouli, sandalwood, tea tree, and vanilla, do not have Mediterranean roots.

Despite the origin of my chosen 20 essential oils, they are now used in European countries, agrees Monika Haas, managing director of the California-based Pacific Institute of Aromatherapy. But she also points out, "where they grow naturally is climate dependent." So, while a handful of the top picks are not exactly originally from the Mediterranean, the majority are and/or are used there.

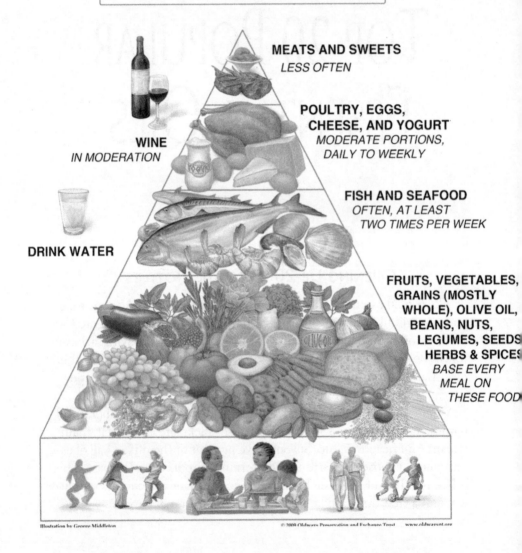

Mediterranean Diet Pyramid

A contemporary approach to delicious, healthy eating

MEATS AND SWEETS
LESS OFTEN

WINE
IN MODERATION

POULTRY, EGGS, CHEESE, AND YOGURT
MODERATE PORTIONS, DAILY TO WEEKLY

FISH AND SEAFOOD
OFTEN, AT LEAST TWO TIMES PER WEEK

DRINK WATER

FRUITS, VEGETABLES, GRAINS (MOSTLY WHOLE), OLIVE OIL, BEANS, NUTS, LEGUMES, SEEDS HERBS & SPICES
BASE EVERY MEAL ON THESE FOOD

Illustration by George Middleton   © 2009 Oldways Preservation and Exchange Trust   www.oldwayspt.org

In fact, the edible essential oils I bring to you are paired with the healthful foods, herbs, and spices included in the Oldways Mediterranean Diet pyramid and chart. Interestingly, the Mediterranean diet was reported in the *U.S. News and World Report* as the best diet to follow in 2019.

Common Foods and Flavors of the Mediterranean Diet Pyramid

Vegetables & Tubers	Artichokes, Arugula, Beets, Broccoli, Brussels Sprouts, Cabbage, Carrots, Celery, Celeriac, Chicory, Collard Cucumber, Dandelion Greens, Eggplant, Fennel, Kale, Leeks, Lettuce, Mache, Mushrooms, Mustard Greens, Nettles, Okra, Onions (red, sweet, white), Peas, Peppers, Potatoes, Pumpkin, Purslane, Radishes, Rutabega, Scallions, Shallots, Spinach, Sweet Potatoes, Turnips, Zucchini
Fruits	Avocados, Apples, Apricots, Cherries, Clementines, Dates, Figs, Grapefruit, Grapes, Lemons, Oranges, Melons, Nectarines, Olives, Peaches, Pears, Pomegranates, Strawberries, Tangerines, Tomatoes
Grains	Breads, Barley, Buckwheat, Bulgur, Couscous, Durum, Farro, Millet, Oats, Polenta, Rice, Wheatberries
Fish & Seafood	Abalone, Cockles, Clams, Crab, Eel, Flounder, Lobster, Mackerel, Mussels, Octopus, Oysters, Salmon, Sardines, Sea Bass, Shrimp, Squid, Tilapia, Tuna, Whelk, Yellowtail
Poultry, Eggs, Cheese, & Yogurt	Chicken, Duck, Guinea Fowl Eggs (Chicken, Quail, and Duck) Cheeses (Examples Include: Brie, Chevre, Corvo, Feta, Haloumi, Manchego, Parmigiano-Reggiano, Pecorino, Ricotta) Yogurt, Greek Yogurt
Nuts, Seeds, & Legumes	Almonds, Beans (Cannellini, Chickpeas, Fava, Kidney, Green), Cashews, Hazelnuts, Lentils, Pine Nuts, Pistachios, Sesame Seeds (Tahini), Split Peas, Walnuts
Herbs & Spices	Anise, Basil, Bay Leaf, Chiles, Clove, Cumin, Fennel, Garlic, Lavender, Marjoram, Mint, Oregano, Parsley, Pepper, Pul Biber, Rosemary, Sage, Savory, Sumac, Tarragon, Thyme, Za'atar
Meats & Sweets	Pork, Beef, Lamb, Mutton, Goat Sweets (Examples include: Baklava, Biscotti, Crème Caramel, Chocolate, Gelato, Fruit Tarts, Kunefe, Lokum, Mousse Au Chocolat, Sorbet, Tiramisu)
Water & Wine	Drink Plenty of Water Wine in Moderation

       www.oldwayspt.org

The Mediterranean Diet is connected to Mediterranean countries, such as Greece, and its people are known to have good health and longevity. The diet includes fruit, vegetables, fish, eggs, nuts, whole grains, some dairy, and olive oil. Also, the well-balanced Mediterranean Diet is celebrated because it is heart-healthy, can help you lose weight, lower your risk of diabetes, and increase longevity. Some scientists give credit to the French paradox, when eating food containing saturated fat does not end up in heart disease or obesity. It may be counteracted by drinking antioxidant-rich red wine; and eating smaller portions of food in contrast to the Western diet. Whatever the reason it works, the fact is—it works!

Take a look at the Oldways Food Chart and Pyramid on the previous pages. I include recipes at the end of chapters (many of these are edible essential oil-infused dishes) and you will discover the last chapter is chock-full of Mediterranean food recipes, with a dash of essential oils for the food menu including breakfast items, appetizers, soups and salads, entrées, and desserts to titillate your nose and palate as well as provide you extra healing compounds and antioxidants for good health and well-being.

Basil

(Ocimum basilicum)

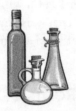

She had no knowledge when day was done,
And the new morn she saw not: but in peace
Hung over her sweet Basil evermore . . .
"For cruel 'tis," said she
"To steal my Basil-pot away from me."
—JOHN KEATS, *Isabella*, st. LIII and LXII

Autumn in San Jose, California, is touted for its Mediterranean climate (a gardener's heaven) and Indian summers. I recall as a kid, outdoor dinners were commonplace and provide fond images of wholesome home-cooked food on the weekends. Our backyard, a refuge for me, was landscaped by my dad and included a small herb and vegetable garden on the side of the house. The garden of life was an oasis for me. The plants produced a potpourri of goodness, including one of my favorites—basil. To create the savory homemade essential oil, my mother would grind fresh basil, dry it, combine it with vegetable oil and sun-dry it for weeks. She then used it in spaghetti and chicken with our home-grown tomatoes.

On an autumn Sunday afternoon, as a fifth grader who loved her English class, I worked on a homework assignment. I remember the aroma from the kitchen was tantalizing.

My mom called out to me, "Come here and taste what is on the stovetop."

She removed the top of the big pot and I sniffed the sweet and spicy aroma of Chicken Caccitore—with a hint of basil oil.

And these days, whenever I get a whiff of basil oil it takes me to a quaint kitchen on that day that was my haven, a place where I read cookbooks and learned about food and aromas.

THE ROOTS OF BASIL

Enter basil. It was first grown in India, and has been grown in the Mediterranean for five thousand years. It is believed the roots of its botanical name—*Ocimum*—is from the Greek word "to smell."

Basil, the herb *and* most likely the oil, is one of the antibacterial herbs used in the legendary blend of Thieves Vinegar, to fight the medieval bubonic plague epidemic. Also, 1500s' herbalist John Gerard wrote that the aroma of basil "taketh away sorrowfulness." Perhaps his keen observance is due to the components in this fragrant herb, which contains many healing powers to help enhance better health.

These days, in the twenty-first century, aromatherapists will tell you basil essential oil is distilled from the leaves and flowering tops. Basil oil is used as a cost-effective ingredient in perfume and soap as well as to flavor Mediterranean dishes. And, you'll discover later on, basil essential oil contains healing secrets that can be used for home cures, too.

BASIL ESSENTIALS

Basil essential oil is a pale-yellow liquid. It is more concentrated and more potent than the fresh, fragrant herb. Healing compounds are found in basil oil, which like most essential oils is steam distilled. Basil essential oil includes basil leaves, stems, and flowering tops.

The three mighty properties in basil oil, noted by researchers in medical studies, are the oxygenated monoterpenes, sesquiterpene hydrocarbons, and sesquiterpenes. Basil oil, not unlike the fresh herb, which I love to use in pesto sauce, is also a good source of disease-fighting antioxidants. The constituents include linalool, 1,8-cinole (eucalyptol), and bergamotene.

MEDICINAL POWERS OF BASIL OIL

Basil oil is believed to help lessen depression, which is a widespread epidemic in the twenty-first century though it can be traced back centuries. Sure, a bout of having the blues can be temporary due to life's stressors, but depression can be a serious illness with many telltale symptoms, including hopelessness, loss of interest in activities, avoiding friends and family, and actually losing interest in day-to-day life.

No, I'm not going to tell you that basil is the latest antidepressant and it will magically put an end to depression. But using basil oil may help lessen negative emotions and unhappy thoughts. It also can help enhance focus and memory as it aids in blood circulation. Its fragrant aroma helps boost alertness, which can help you stay in the present rather than dwell on "what if's" in the future.[1] And there's more to this super powerful antidepressant essential oil that you should know about . . . According to findings at the Indian Council of Medical Research, basil essential oil has also been used as treatment for respiratory infections and kidney problems. Thanks to the potent bacteria-fighting compounds methyl eugenol and methychavicolis, basil oil is a healing wonder.[2]

Additional Advantages: Basil essential oil has many therapeutic benefits, from aiding in digestive woes to fighting viruses such as the common cold and flu. Headaches (all types from tension to sinus) may go away with basil oil, and it may also help boost energy and lessen fatigue, too. It is touted as a natural cough suppressant and can even help heal some skin conditions.

Come On, Try It! Basil oil is often inhaled to enjoy its healing benefits. You can use it in a diffuser, vaporizer, or sniff it out of a vial for fast relief. It can also be found in a cream or lotion and used topically. It is an aromatic and flavorful culinary essential oil, and as I can personally attest, it works well in Mediterranean food recipes.

Essential Safety Tip: It should be avoided during pregnancy.

Healing
Basil Pesto Pasta

This basil pesto pasta, a scrumptious dish whose roots go way back to the ancient Roman era, is a favorite dish of mine. Pesto salad is nothing new, but mint oil can give it a new kick and tomatoes always go with basil. This pasta can be a side dish or a main dish and is good served hot or cold. This recipe is inspired by my godmother, a Pioneer Woman–type wizard in the kitchen, who served it to me for the first time when I was kid with an unsophisticated palate. The long noodles mixed with a distinct taste of basil oil makes it a dish you can savor year-round if you don't have access to the fresh herb.

1 cup fresh basil leaves
½ clove garlic
Ground pepper and sea salt to taste
¼ cup pine nuts (optional toast in oven)
¼ cup extra virgin olive oil
1 drop basil oil
2 cups whole grain pasta, cooked (spaghetti or rotini, preferred)
¼ cup Parmesan cheese, shavings
Fresh parsley sprigs
¼ cup Roma tomatoes, sliced, garnish (optional)

In a food processor or blender, chop and puree basil, garlic, pepper, and salt. Add nuts, olive oil, and basil oil. Set aside. Boil pasta in a large pot of water and drain it carefully. Top ½ cup pesto sauce on 1 cup hot pasta. Toss with pasta or leave on top. Sprinkle with cheese. Garnish with parsley and tomatoes. Add fresh and warm French bread or baguette slices either dipped in olive oil or spread with European-style butter.

Serves 2 to 4.

Now that you're aware of the powers of basil oil, I'll show you how cedarwood—a woodsy essential oil available for centuries, continues to get attention from aromatherapists, researchers, consumers, and me. It's the memories of cedar from my childhood and young adult years that are heartfelt—and this essential oil may be added to your choice of favored oils, too.

SCENT-SATIONAL HEALING OILS SHORT & SWEET

✓ Basil essential oil contains plenty of nutrients, including the compounds monoterpenes and sesquiterpenes, that can enhance brainpower and blood flow to feel energized and alive!
✓ Consider using basil essential oil with its potent bacteria-fighting compounds methyl eugenol and methychavicolis, especially during cold and flu season.
✓ Get innovative! Combine fresh basil for texture and presentation *and* a tiny bit of basil essential oil for flavor.
✓ Remember, use only a droplet to make nutrient-dense foods even more delicious and healthful. (Refer to the recipes chapter.)
✓ Adding basil essential oil to edible recipes, paired with heart-healthy Mediterranean Diet staples such as vegetables and whole grains, will give you extra antioxidants, especially if added last to a dish to preserve the nutrients.

Cedarwood

(Cedrus atlantica)

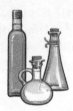

Cedar, and pine, and fir, and branching palm,
A sylvan scene, and, as the ranks ascend
Shade above shade, a woody theatre
Of stateliest view.
—JOHN MILTON, *Paradise Lost*, Bk. IV

At twelve, I was an awkward teenager most comfortable solo and in the company of my dog and nature. On one weekend, I recall my older sister, popular and prettier than me, was out at the beach with her friends and I was alone with my canine pal in our bedroom. She had a personal locked cedar hope chest with a strong woodsy sweet aroma. I did pry it open. But unlike Pandora's box, the contents were cedar scented (she used the cedarwood essential oil to maintain its fragrance). The items included lingerie, household linens, crystal glasses, and china—stuff a woman keeps in anticipation of marriage. I was envious of the rich woodsy aroma–scented cedarwood box of promise.

Years later, when we led our separate lives, I didn't marry but I did have a beloved dog. Sadly, my eleven-year-old black Labrador with brown soulful eyes whom I hitched and hiked across America with had died abruptly from kidney disease. His ashes were put into a small cedarwood box. When traveling soon after his passing on a business trip I took the box with me; and because I had slept with my loyal canine companion for more than a decade, I slipped the box under the covers with me in the sterile hotel room. The sweet, woodsy scent of the reddish-brown-colored cedar box made me feel warm and comforted despite the loss and my grieving for woman's best friend who protected me.

THE ROOTS OF CEDARWOOD

So cedarwood has an unforgettable history with me but its roots are much older. The almighty cedar tree, noted in the Bible, can be as tall as one hundred feet and its life span can be more than a thousand years. Cedarwood was believed to be used for embalming the deceased more than five thousand years ago. It was noted on a Babylonian tablet in 1800 B.C. that caretakers of the sick cleared toxic energy, treated people with leprosy and skin disorders with cedarwood oil. These medicines and the calming effects of cedar oil all go back to ancient uses.[1]

Historians believe cedarwood was used to build temples, including one for King Solomon. People thought the cedar aroma would connect worshippers closer to God. Centuries ago, the Sumerians and Egyptians used cedar oil from the Cedar of Leamnon for embalming the deceased.

Like basil oil, cedarwood—also called cedar—has a strong scent, but this oil is richer and woodsier, which is appealing to the nose. In the 1970s, the trend of using cedarwood saunas in health clubs, bathhouses, hotels, and homes was popular. Cedarwood is still a common wood you'll find in a sauna—a small, heated room that people use to relax and sweat for health's sake. Cedarwood oil can be used in medicine, perfume, aromatherapy blends, and even as an insecticide because of its powerful components.

CEDARWOOD ESSENTIALS

Surprise! There are different species, not just one, of cedarwood. Atlas and Himalayan are from the cedar genus and Virginia and Texas varieties are from the Juniper genus. The thing is, all types of cedarwood oil contain sesquiterpenes. The Juniper cedarwood includes cedrol and thujopsene. It's the cedrol and cedrane, however, which help to produce the rich balsamic odor.

Unlike basil essential oil, cedarwood oil is extracted from wood—but the extraction method is also steam distillation. Scented cedar oil is not used as a culinary essential oil, but it does contain healing properties that can be used for a wide range of medicinal and therapeutic purposes. As noted in the ORAC chart in chapter 1, cedarwood oil ranks high on the disease-fighting antioxidant list among essential oils.

MEDICINAL POWERS OF CEDARWOOD OIL

The sweet and nutty scented cedarwood with its wide variety of compounds provides healing powers such as an anti-inflammatory, antiseptic, as well as a sedative for calming nerves. Perhaps the most intriguing benefit of cedarwood oil is its immunity-enhancing powers.

Cedarwood oil is believed to have the potential ability to fight leukemia cells, according to research at a Lebanese university. It was discovered that cedarwood oil may be useful in inhibiting drug-resistant tumors. The jury is still out on giving definitive credit to cedarwood as a proven cancer fighter, but some people who are looking for nature's alternatives may be tempted to give it a try, especially if their cancer is in remission, stage one and slow growing, or just as an anti-cancer preventative measure to include in a healthful diet and lifestyle.[2]

Additional Advantages: Cedarwood oil may also help in staving off respiratory viruses and toxic environmental pollutions that can lead to infections and lung or sinus congestion. It is effective for different health ailments, including aiding in depression, preventing respiratory infections, heart disease, and lessening inflammation in some skin conditions. Cedarwood is also an excellent insect repellant, which I use. (Refer to chapter 27 for outdoor household information of essential oils.)

Come On, Try It! Using an aromatic vaporizer with cedarwood oil is one method that works to get its healing effects. I have splashed water on the hot rocks in a cedarwood sauna to get more of the warm scent to clear my sinuses and congestion during the wintertime. Cedarwood oil can also be used diluted with water or added to a non-scented lotion for skin conditions like acne and insect stings or bites.

Essential Safety Tip: Cedar fragrance should be avoided during pregnancy due to its possible powerful stimulant and sedative effects.

Destressing
Cedar Orange Perfume

❖ ❖ ❖

This recipe is inspired by my love for California (aka the Golden State) and its woodsy aromas, like cedarwood saunas and orange trees, a year-round citrus fruit grown in the suburbs of San Jose, once an agricultural paradise. As a youngster, I'd climb on the cedarwood fence my father built to pick ripe oranges from the neighbor's tree after taking a dip in their swimming pool. This down-to-earth perfume mix—including cedarwood oil and orange oil—is close to my heart because it triggers memories of nature's wood, water, fruit, and fun, during the carefree days of my adventurous youth.

3 drops orange oil
2 drops cedarwood oil
1 drop jasmine absolute
6 drops sandalwood oil
10 ml jojoba oil

Blend essential oils with 10 mL jojoba oil as the carrier oil. Put a dab on your wrist, chest, or neck.

In the next chapter, I'll introduce you to chamomile—yes chamomile, my favorite herbal tea and essential oil. You may already love it or you will after I show you how much you can do with it. Take a look at intriguing findings, from the past and present, and you, like me, can discover how to use chamomile essential oil.

SCENT-SATIONAL HEALING OILS SHORT & SWEET

✓ Sniffing the aroma of cedarwood with its disease-fighting antioxidants may help bolster the immune system, lower the risk of stress, colds, or even respiratory infections.

✓ Cedar contains a host of antioxidants, which makes it a functional oil that you can benefit from in non-edible ways unlike culinary basil essential oil.

✓ Listen up when aromatherapists tout cedar oil for its therapeutic usage in aromatherapeutic massage, inhaling the oil used in diffusers, perfumes, incense, and even baths.

✓ Don't forget cedarwood oil with its strong scent and bacteria-fighting properties is a good essential oil to use in aromatic blends for both medicinal and therapeutic healing powers.

Chamomile

(Matricaria recutita)

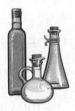

*The Camomile; the more of it is troden on, the faster it
grows.*
—WILLIAM SHAKESPEARE, *Henry IV, Part 1*,
Act 2, Scene 4

Fast forward to another aromatherapy fragrant herb introduced to me
when I was at that self-conscious tween age. Hello chamomile. One
weekend my grandmother, a retired English teacher from the desert in
Arizona, visited us. My mother and father would say, "She's too eccen-
tric," but I adored her. One Saturday night she filled up the tub (this
was our routine) but this time she put a special herbal oil concoction
into the bubble bath. The water was filled up to the very top, not
halfway like I was used to during the water rationing due to a past
drought. In the bathroom she served me macaroons and a small cup of
chamomile tea.

Then, she asked me what story I'd like to hear.

I said, "I love white fluffy bunny rabbits."

So she chose to read Beatrix Potter's *The Tale of Peter Rabbit*. She explained to me that when he came home, his mother gave him a tablespoon of chamomile tea to help him relax and go to sleep. This comforting story paired with an aromatic bath and treats was unforgettable and bonded me to my gran, who later became an influence in my own adventures on the road, including a hitchhiking trip through the desert to visit her and getting much needed guidance in my early twenties.

THE ROOTS OF CHAMOMILE

For more than two thousand years, chamomile has been considered a healing plant, which is extracted to give us the powerful essential oil. It was called "ground apple" by the Greeks because of its fragrant smell, like fresh apples off a tree.

The Egyptians believed chamomile to be sacred to the sun god Ra. The petals, which are the essence of the soothing essential oil, were also added to the baths of royalty to help them calm down and sleep.

Ancient chamomile oil comes from the flowers of the plant, which looks similar to the simple but elegant white and yellow daisy. The popular and versatile essential oil is made by steam distillation of the flower dried in the sunshine for a short spell.

CHAMOMILE ESSENTIALS

The fact is, there are two varieties of chamomile oil: Roman (*Anthemis nobilis*) is believed by aromatherapy gurus to be more calming. The collection method of the oil is taken from the flower and extracted through steam distillation. It contains 1,8 cinole, phenolic acids, and tannins. German chamomile oil can also help you to relax, but it works better as a potent anti-inflammatory oil thanks to its compound azulene.[1] But that's not all . . .

It's the terpenoids and flavonoids such as apigenin that provide the therapeutic cosmetic and nutritional benefits of chamomile essential oil. This flavonoid, which has antioxidant properties, may inhibit the growth of skin tumors. But more research is needed before chamomile oil can be labeled as a cancer fighter.

Chamomile oil provides both a sweet and mild subtle scent. Sure, chamomile oil is a super source of components that are excellent for calming your nervous system. But it does so much more.

MEDICINAL POWERS OF CHAMOMILE OIL

Chamomile essential oil, much like the chamomile tea I love and sip daily, can have the same positive effects on keeping blood pressure in a healthy numbers range. When pressure is used on blood vessels and arteries, it causes pressure on your heart, which can up the odds of heart attack or stroke. Some causes of increasing normal blood pressure include emotional stress.

Using chamomile oil can help lower the blood pressure numbers. It works by lowering stress levels, which can help to dilate your arteries. And antioxidants, which we know are in the oil, lower oxidative stress. Both types of chamomile can lower blood pressure and the swelling of blood vessels. Also, chamomile is a nervine, which can help to maintain the nervous system and keep you calmer.

Research shows when chamomile essential oil vapors are inhaled it can help to lessen stress. For this reason it is nature's blood pressure medicine. We know high blood pressure can lead to heart disease, diabetes, and other health ailments—which makes chamomile essential oil a must-have to help stay chill.

Chamomile soap infused with essential oils is available in the guest rooms at the Southern California spa Cal-a-Vie. The spa director praises the natural organic item. "It helps to relieve acne, burns, cuts, insect bites, rashes, and wounds."

Additional Advantages: The healing uses of Roman chamomile are varied, but some important ones I personally love are its ability to stave off anxiety, depression, insomnia, and stress. Often, these mental disorders overlap. They can be short term and/or chronic and linger on—either way chamomile essential oil can be helpful. Chamomile oil can calm pre-menstrual crankies, cramps, and cravings because it can relax tense muscles.

It is known to be used as an anti-anxiety healing oil similar to chamomile tea, my all-time favorite herbal beverage; and its sweet and mild scent is like the welcoming fragrance of the "friendliest flower" as Meg Ryan's character called it in my favorite romantic comedy *You've Got Mail*.

Come On, Try It! Chamomile oil can be used topically, sniffed, or consumed. It can also be used in calming baths and massages, and inhaled from a vial or in a vaporizer. This essential oil is also infused in a variety of products, including beauty, cleaning, and personal hygiene from soaps to shampoos. Whether it's a spray for the air or put into an aromatherapy necklace that you can wear for its calming benefits, like I do, it's one essential oil that is essential to me and may be for you, too.

Calming and Healing Chamomile-Infused Oatmeal and Honey Facial Mask

Imagine making an at-home easy to use all-purpose mask to soothe and soften skin. Living in a dry climate your skin may lack hydration, like mine does, thanks to the lack of humidity in the Sierra of Northern California. Here is a facial with healing foods you likely have in your refrigerator and pantry. Go ahead—brew a cup of chamomile tea and put together this recipe for a beautifying scent-sation that's perfect for dry skin.

1 cup rolled oats
½ cup plain yogurt
1 teaspoon honey
1 egg white
1 drop essential almond oil, sweet
1 drop chamomile essential oil

In a food processor or blender, process oatmeal until finely ground. Add the remaining ingredients and process until mixed well. Apply to neck and face in circular motions. Leave on skin for 10 to 15 minutes. Remove with warm water. Can be applied once per week. Must make a fresh batch each time.

(Courtesy: LorAnn Oils)

Speaking of chamomile bliss, you may also cherish the next essential oil with a bit more of a kick. Cinnamon is a popular spice and the oil is a keeper. Turn the pages ahead to find out exactly why cinnamon goes far beyond the kitchen and is useful for healing the mind, body, and spirit year-round in every room in your home.

SCENT-SATIONAL HEALING OILS SHORT & SWEET

✓ If you're prone to feeling the scourge of high stress, Roman chamomile oil, thanks to its calming components, such as 1,8 cinole, flavonoids, phenolic acids, and tannins, may help you to chill . . .
✓ Be aware that stress can be connected to colds, flu, and even cancer since it can weaken the immune system, but chamomile oil can provide protection so you're less vulnerable.
✓ Learn to recognize when your blood pressure numbers spike because taking a whiff of chamomile oil or a rub with chamomile oil can aid in keeping those numbers in check. (Refer to the anti-aging chapter.)
✓ Chamomile, a mild essential oil thanks to its terpenoids and flavonoids, such as apigenin, provides therapeutic uses for skin care, from cuts and abrasions to dry skin.
✓ Chamomile oil is often paired with other essential oils when used in beauty creations and DIY blends for the skin and hair. It is a common oil since it is gentle, unlike other more potent essential oils . . .
✓ Don't forget to check out recipes that include food-grade chamomile essential oil. It is commonly used in hot water for tea or as an ingredient in baked goods, including scones, cakes, and cookies because it has a mild, sweet flavor and calming benefits, too.

Cinnamon

(*Cinnamomum zeylanicum*)

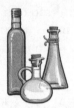

*We make conquest only of husks and shells for the
most part—at least apparently,—but sometimes
these are cinnamon and spices, you know.*
—HENRY DAVID THOREAU,
    letter to Richard Fuller, 1843

Before leaving my unexciting home in suburbia, cinnamon oil made its
way into my sheltered world, too. Memories of cinnamon rolls one
Sunday linger in my mind, and often the spice takes me back to the
suburbs on a particular overcast autumn morning. It was my sixteenth
birthday. I was dealing with the challenge of being friendless in a new
high school and coping with Tin Man braces. After I was fitted with
the metal contraption—my teeth felt like buttes and my mouth ached.

"I look like a *Twilight Zone* monster," I mumbled when I passed on
eating breakfast.

My dad, a strong and stoic war veteran who received a purple heart,
said, "Your smile will be beautiful. Stay strong."

His words made me feel warm and fuzzy, as did the aroma of the zesty cinnamon rolls infused with cinnamon oil baking in the oven my mother had made from scratch. They tasted sweet and spicy and made me feel good and safe at home.

Dishing out sweet and spicy cinnamon rolls takes me back in time to 2006. I was on a book tour with the late geologist Jim Berkland, a surrogate father figure. After a long day of back-to-back bookstore signings in the San Francisco Bay area, it was back home to his Glen Ellen house, a nature lover's paradise. I retreated to the guest room, which had a rustic charm. In my purse, I had a packaged cinnamon roll from the airport. It was not homemade but it was doable. I found a box of essential oils in the bathroom cupboard. I chose cinnamon oil and put one drop mixed with an almond oil onto my hands. The oil combination gave my bath an earthy fragrance. I destressed from the busy day and felt at home.

These days, I use cinnamon in many forms (ground, fresh sticks, incense, and essential oil). Its multipurpose merits are remarkable. It's time to share what I've discovered—you will want to earmark this info for your daily life.

Ode to Birds, Snakes, and Cinnamon Bark

As the legend goes, cinnamon bark, which provides the spicy essential oil when extracted, was a luxury centuries ago because it was a hardship to obtain it. One tale occurred during the fifth-century B.C. as told by Greek historian Herodotus. It was said that huge birds carried cinnamon sticks to their nests high on mountains, a place where humans could not go. So savvy individuals would leave ox meat on the ground for the birds. When the creatures brought the meat up to the nests the weight would cause the nests to drop and then the cinnamon could be picked up.

A more challenging cinnamon tale is the one where the spice was found in canyons surrounded by snakes. It was only the brave who would travel on rafts to glean the spice and travel far to deliver the goods to people who appreciated it and how it was brought to them, according to the Greek philosopher Pliny who shared the tale. As time passed, cinnamon was easier to obtain, and in present-day cinnamon oil is one of the most popular essential oils.

THE ROOTS OF CINNAMON

Cinnamon oil is a warming spice, a favorite aroma in autumn and winter. Cinnamon comes from a big reddish-brown tree with scented bark that is grown in subtropical regions and is cultivated in Indonesia and China.

This dark colored essential oil, like most of the twenty oils I chose, is made by the distillation method using both the leaves and bark. In the twentieth century, Yardley's produced a fragrant soap with flecks of cinnamon, which was one I used and loved as a teenager.

CINNAMON ESSENTIALS

One of the most antioxidant-rich essential oils is cinnamon oil. The cassia type from the leaf is less expensive, whereas the Ceylon variety from the bark is very potent and very pricey and not used often. Cinnamon leaf essential oil is steam distilled from the leaf and bark, and contains eugenol and cinnamaldehyde. Cinnamon bark essential oil is steam distilled only from the bark. It has less eugenol and more cinnamaldehyde.

Cinnamon essential oil also boasts phenols, compounds that act as powerful antioxidants that protect your body by trapping free radical molecules before damage happens. (Refer to the ORAC chart in chapter 1.) It's these almighty phenols that are believed to stave off viruses and bacteria, which often can lead to health ailments like a cold or bad cholesterol and even life-threatening diseases, such as cancer and heart disease.

But note, other healing compounds in cinnamon oil include a-cedrene, cedrol, thujopsene, camphor, and linalool, the Zen calm ingredient.

MEDICINAL POWERS OF CINNAMON OIL

Cinnamon oil is given credit for providing many health benefits, including decreasing LDL or "bad" cholesterol and improving heart health. Small studies have shown cinnamon oil contain an anti-inflammatory thanks to phenylpropanoid. This, in result, means that it may help with anti-plaque effect so your arteries won't be clogged leading to heart disease. More research is needed.

Not only is cinnamon oil good for your heart, but past research has also shown that because of its multitude of compounds it may be helpful for keeping your blood sugar levels on an even keel. In one study published in *Diabetes Care*, sixty people with type 2 diabetes were given three different amounts of cinnamon in capsules. After forty days there was a decrease in their blood sugar *and* triglycerides, LDL "bad" cholesterol, and total cholesterol. This, in turn, means adding a bit of cinnamon essential oil to a healthful diet may help you stave off unsteady sugar levels and/or diabetes.[1]

Researchers have discovered the therapeutic effects of cinnamon's scent, which is also in the linalool-rich essential oil which can be calming, and even may lessen pain. Studies show that the oil can help to relax tight muscles, which can benefit painful joints and boost blood circulation.

Also, this powerful essential oil with its eugenol compound may help stave off viral, fungal, and bacterial infections as it can boost the immune system, thanks to its antioxidant power.

Additional Advantages: Cinnamon oil enhances mental and physical well-being, too. It is also known for its "sexual healing," with respect to the classic Marvin Gaye's song title, and it may be due to its ability to stimulate blood circulation. The aroma of cinnamon rolls or cookies can induce memories of childhood. It can give you a warm feeling, which is due to the limbic system that triggers emotions in the brain, you know that feel-good scent that takes you to a happy place.

Come On, Try It! There are many ways to use cinnamon oil, which include inhaling it from a vial, diffuser, or applying it directly to the skin with a carrier oil, especially if you have sensitive skin. Cinnamon oil is also a popular culinary essential oil used in both cooking and baking.

The first time I was introduced to the oil was from King Arthur Flour company. I was hesitant to use it since ground cinnamon was my normal—but I tried it. And I'm glad I did.

Not only does the oil provide extra flavor to baked goods, the scent transports you to a world of autumn goodness, a time of fresh, crisp air and fragrant spice scents of the season. Cinnamon oil adds extra flavor to a smoothie or even tea. This warming oil can also be used diluted with water as a compress on your body to soothe achy muscles and cramps. Cinnamon oil is a versatile essential oil that has an infinite number of uses.

Essential Safety Tip: It is a potent oil so dilute it with a carrier oil or water when bathing or using a compress to avoid irritation.

Mood-Enhancing Cinnamon Rolls

This recipe will rock your taste buds like it does mine. I paired the cinnamon rolls with my own essential oil touch to give an extra cinnamon punch to the vanilla glaze, which will whisk you away to your comfort zone.

DOUGH

½ cup milk
1 tablespoon dry yeast
1 egg (or 2 egg whites)
1 teaspoon vanilla extract
3 tablespoons Marsala Olive Fruit Oil
2 cups flour
2 tablespoons semolina
½ teaspoon salt
⅓ cup sugar

FILLING

4 to 5 tablespoons brown sugar
1¼ teaspoons cinnamon
¼ teaspoon cardamom
½ cup raisin, dried blueberries, or cherries
3 to 4 teaspoons Marsala Olive Fruit Oil

In a mixing bowl add milk and yeast, let stand about 10 minutes. Stir in egg, vanilla, and oil. Add remaining ingredients, stir until dough holds together. Cover, let rise in a warm place until doubled, about 1 hour. Turn dough out onto floured board, pat dough down to 12-by-8 inch rectangle. Brush with olive oil, sprinkle with remaining ingredients evenly. Moisten edges, roll dough up jelly-roll style, beginning with long end. Slice roll with heavy thread, placing under roll. Crisscross thread across top of roll, pulling quickly as if tying a knot. Place rolls cut side up in a 10-inch greased baking pan. Leave a little space in between rolls. Let stand covered in a warm place until puffy, about 1 hour. Bake at 375 degrees F for 25 to 35 minutes, or until golden. Cover with foil loosely if browning too quickly. [Author's note: See my glaze recipe below.]

Makes 12.

(Courtesy: Gemma Sanita Sciabica, *Baking with California Olive Oil: Dolci and Biscotti Recipes*)

CINNAMON GLAZE

½ cup confectioners sugar
2 tablespoons organic half-and-half
½ teaspoon vanilla extract
1 drop cinnamon essential oil

In a small bowl mix sugar, half-and-half, vanilla, and oil until smooth. Drizzle glaze on top of cooled rolls. These rolls are ideal for breakfast, brunch, a snack or dessert.

Loving cinnamon oil is not a difficult task for most people. After all, the aroma often lingers in the kitchen during and after baking. Moving along in the wide world of essential oils, another therapeutic pick of mine is eucalyptus. Get ready to meet an essential oil that has its roots in yesteryear. Not only is its aroma breathtaking (literally), it boasts benefits for your body and health.

SCENT-SATIONAL HEALING OILS SHORT & SWEET

✓ Remember, one of the most antioxidant-rich essential oils is cinnamon oil. The bark variety is more potent. This essential oil boasts phenols, compounds that act as powerful antioxidants that protect your body by trapping free radical molecules before damage happens. (Refer to the ORAC chart in chapter 1.)

✓ It's these almighty phenols that are believed to stave off viruses and bacteria, which often can lead to health ailments like a cold or bad cholesterol and even life-threatening diseases, such as cancer and heart disease.

✓ Don't forget, other healing compounds in essential cinnamon oil like linalool can provide calming effects to your mind and body.

✓ Jot down the fact that the anti-inflammatory phenylpropanoid in the essential oil may help stave off plaque and clogged arteries.

✓ If you or someone you know is coping with lowering triglycerides as well as blood sugar levels, including cinnamon essential oil in a heart-healthy lifestyle may help to get those numbers on an even keel.

✓ Psst! If you're trying to lose unwanted weight, essential cinnamon oil can help. (Refer to "The Slimming Essentials" chapter to find out how it works.)

✓ Cinnamon oil isn't just a warming aroma for autumn and winter . . . think outside of the spice rack and use the spicy essential oil all year long for better health and well-being.

Eucalyptus

(Eucalyptus globulus and Eucalyptus radiata)

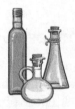

*The tall eucalyptus walked along the valley of
dreamers and spoke among a throng of almond and
olives and told of days that no man sees.*
—ALTAIR LAAHAD, *Eucalyptus Talk*

Eucalyptus is more of a medicinal herbal oil and like other essential oils I've shared with you, comes with feel-good memories. Images of eucalyptus trees in Monterey, a coastal town cloaked in fog that lies along the Pacific Ocean, come to me each time I use this fragrant essential oil. But eucalyptus oil is more than just an extraordinary breathtaking tree; it allows you to breathe easy. As a young teen, one school week I came home on a rainy, winter day. I complained of the all-too-common sore throat you get before a cold sets in. The next morning, I had a chest cold, was congested with "gookies" in the throat, and a runny nose soon followed. During the illness, my mom treated me with nature's remedies.

This included lots of bed rest, hot chicken soup, orange juice, and one oh-so smelly over-the-counter product called Vicks VapoRub. It was a popular topical chest rub ointment that came with a strong scent. As I grew up, I discovered its ingredients include oil of eucalyptus, cedar leaf, and nutmeg oil. While I didn't like the pungent odor, or greasy feel on my chest, I admit it did help me breathe and sleep better through the night. It was my mother's little helper and worked like a charm.

THE ROOTS OF EUCALYPTUS

As aromatherapy historians will tell you, for thousands of years, people have used the strong-smelling and almost overpowering eucalyptus oil. It was believed the eucalyptus tree was health-giving because it purified the natural environment. People with health ailments often migrated to regions where the tree grew to heal. The parts used to extract the essential oil are part of the tree trunk, leaves, stems, and twigs. It is extracted through steam distillation.

The beautiful eucalyptus tree was exported to the Mediterranean countries as well as throughout the world, growing best in Mediterranean climates, like what I experienced as a kid in the suburbs of San Jose.

Aromatherapists will tell you the tree was first noticed centuries ago, but the oil was first distilled in Australia in the mid-nineteenth century. By the early twentieth century eucalyptus oil was produced for profit in Australia because its medicinal magic was believed to have therapeutic effects.

EUCALYPTUS ESSENTIALS

There are two varieties of eucalyptus oil, the *globulus* and *radiata*. The eucalyptus globulus is more potent, whereas the radiata is more gentle. The essential oil has a powerful but stimulating intense fragrance, but it's refreshing once accustomed to it.

The primary healing component of eucalyptus essential oil is eucalyptol (1,8-cinole). You can find this ingredient listed in a store-bought essential oil or in ointments used in vapor rubs for respiratory ailments. Cinole is an anti-inflammatory and is used in inhalants, ointments, and lozenges that boast antibacterial benefits. Other main constituents include a (alpha)-pinene, and limonene.

MEDICINAL POWERS OF EUCALYPTUS OIL

It is no shocker that eucalyptus oil has a wide variety of proven healing benefits backed up by both anecdotal reports and scientific research. It is touted for its ability to keep at bay respiratory infections and even sinusitis—a blasted ailment I've had since I was a kid and pops up after a long airline flight and during the wintertime.

Eucalyptus oil is one of the best essential oils to help keep the flu at bay because it apparently boosts your body's immune system. Dr. Kurt Schnaubelt, founder of the Pacific Aromatherapy Institute points, out that "the most effective essential oils for viral infections are those with sizable contents of cinole, mono terpene alcohol, and mono terpene hydrocarbons." He adds, "These three types of components form an effective antiviral synergy."

Bronchitis, which is a viral health ailment that can be contagious, too, can be made less severe and recovery may be quicker if one inhales eucalyptus oil. Research shows that eucalyptus oil may be helpful because of its antiviral and antimicrobial properties thanks to its cinole property.[1]

In my thirties when I was a struggling graduate student without health insurance, I experienced bronchitis. Each time I coughed my chest ached. I decided to use a natural remedy. I mixed six drops of eucalyptus oil into a large pot of very hot water. I covered my head with a lightweight towel and inhaled the steam for a few minutes. I was cough-free within one week.

Additional Advantages: The main healing component eucalyptol is also helpful in soothing sore muscles. I can personally attest that it works. By adding a few drops of eucalyptus oil into an all-natural, unscented lotion I rubbed it on my rib cage after overdoing it with too many laps of the breaststroke in the resort swimming pool. The result? I enjoyed instant relief from the achy muscles. I keep a small jar of the miracle worker cream in my medicine cabinet. Not to forget it boasts antiseptic and antiviral benefits. (Refer to the chapter on home cures to find out what DIY remedies you can put to work and use year-round.)

Come On, Try It! So if I've intrigued you with the healing powers of eucalyptus essential oil, you'll be pleased to know that it can be used in aromatic massages, baths and showers, saunas and steams, inhalation from the bottle, put in aromatherapy jewelry, and a vaporizer. It is often used in lotions and salves for its soothing benefits for the body. Eucalyptus oil is an ingredient in some cough medications. Eucalyptus also can help clear sinuses quick by inhaling the aroma by sniffing it from a vial.

Essential Safety Tip: Eucalyptus has varied healing powers but sorry, it is not an edible essential oil.

Rejuvenating
Eucalyptus Body Oil

❖ ❖ ❖

As a tree hugger from the seventies, you'd think I'd love to get all-natural massages with an oil that comes from a eucalyptus tree. Not so much. However, self-massaging with oils after bathing is invigorating and addictive. Eucalyptus massage oil is super for sore or aching muscles due to straining from work or play, a flu bug, or even a hangover. One winter in the Sierra we got minimal snow until one weekend when a late spring snowstorm blanketed the town. On this particular weekend, I was scheduled for a book signing in Reno. Before I left I had to shovel the deck and pathways. Not to forget walk the dog. Upon arriving home, there was more shoveling to be done. This recipe is one I used to soothe my aching muscles and it worked like a charm.

20 drops eucalyptus essential oil
20 drops lavender essential oil
20 drops rose essential oil
5 drops peppermint essential oil
3 ounces almond oil

Add only 30 drops of this blend to three ounces of almond oil or an unscented lotion. Shake and apply on your achy muscles.

Now that you get eucalyptus oil can be as fragrant and refreshing as the leaves in a sauna or inhaling the trees along the road in the Golden State, it's time for me to introduce you to another essential oil—geranium. In the next chapter I'll show you how the perhaps less popular floral oil is a winner among aromatherapists and may win you over, too.

Scent-sational Healing Oils Short & Sweet

✓ Note that the top healing component of eucalyptus essential oil is eucalyptol, which can helps stave off respiratory ailments.
✓ Do understand that eucalyptus essential oil has antibacterial components, such as the cinole compound, which is used in store-bought medicines that can help you fight off irksome germs.
✓ Be mindful of the aromatherapy benefits of this strong oil, often used in saunas to give instant relief for respiratory symptoms, including clearing mucus and coughing.
✓ Keep in mind, you can reduce painful muscles and joints by using oh-so soothing eucalyptus oil because the healing component eucalyptol works as an anti-inflammatory in a bottle!
✓ Follow your instincts. If you feel the ancient-day eucalyptus oil is giving you relief but scientists can't give you a hard-hitting double-blind study for, use your head *and* a eucalyptus oil folk remedy if it works for you.

8

Geranium

(Pelargonium graveoloens)

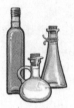

Perfumes are the feelings of flowers.
—HEINRICH HEINE

Geranium oil comes from exotic flowers and it has a pleasant rose-citrus type of floral, woodsy scent unlike the pungent eucalyptus oil aroma. As a teenager, keeping up with my outgoing peers and fads was a task that I tried to master but needed help. The popular scent advertised on TV that was modest in price was Heaven Scent, but wearing the perfume didn't draw attention or make me feel like a confident angel on Earth. Things changed.

A forward-thinking high school friend of my sister's didn't go for the store-bought perfumes from heaven. At all. One day in her bedroom, she brought out a small box. Inside it was a collection of essential oil vials. One was her favorite self-made blend, including earthy peppermint, camphor, bergamot, rosemary, basil—and geranium. She gave it to me as a belated birthday present. It was the gift of my entry into the magical world of aromatic oils to use as personalized perfumes to make me enjoy feeling different and embrace individuality. The flowery geranium oil was unique to me. Its special scent enlivened my passion as an awkward teenager because the alluring scent made me feel confident and grown up.

THE ROOTS OF GERANIUM

The consensus of historical reports about the roots of geranium is that the flower goes back hundreds of years. The floral fragrance of the essential oil is a combination of citrus notes and a woodsy scent. The essential oil presents a delightful aroma like smelling late-blooming springtime flowers in the Sierra Nevada.

Aromatherapists will tell you that geranium oil goes way, way back in time to Bulgaria. It got some recognition by the Thracians, a group of tribes that ruled the Balkans during the Roman era.

GERANIUM ESSENTIALS

Geranium essential oil has a greenish color and is packed with a variety of components. This exotic essential oil is extracted from the sweet flowers and leaves of the plant, using the steam distillation method. One of the main components in this essential oil is geraniol. Other properties in this sweet fragrant oil include citronellol, citral, eugenol, geraniol, linalool, methone, sabine, and terpineol.

It's the mix of these compounds, some, like eugenol, you will notice are found in other essential oils, that are responsible for geranium oil's medicinal and healing powers for the mind and body.

MEDICINAL POWERS OF GERANIUM OIL

Like other essential oils, there isn't one perk to geranium but a wide variety of benefits. Researchers pinpoint the compound geraniol as one property that makes geranium essential oil act like a natural antidepressant and helps ground you while coping with hectic events. We know stress and depression can elevate the odds of developing heart disease and even cancer. But using geranium oil may help in lowering stress levels.

The flowery oil with its eugenol, like eucalyptus, helps fight off inflammation to infections, too. This oil can help beat bacteria and stave off contracting viruses. That means it can help lower your risk of contracting a cold or flu, two conditions that can wreak havoc on your life because it interrupts work and play. But using geranium oil does much more for your well-being, too.

Additional Advantages: Geranium oil is also known for its ability to help cope with a myriad of female-related issues, from painful endometriosis, which I may have had but was never tested to find out for sure, to the scourge of pre-menstrual symptoms that affect millions of women during their childbearing years from teens to fifties. Geranium is believed to rejuvenate your body due to its anti-inflammatory and calming compounds.

Come On, Try It! You can inhale flowery geranium oil from the vial. Or try putting one drop of the floral oil mixed with one drop of a carrier oil like almond oil or jojoba oil on your wrist. Also, you can add geranium oil in a bathtub blend of other essential oils, and a massage cream. It can be used in a vaporizer for inhalation benefits.

Calming Massage Oil
Geranium Recipe

❖ ❖ ❖

In my twenties, I found myself meeting a youthful, charming man with soulful green eyes, wit, and a moving smile at the airport when I was selling handcrafted wooden birds. He worked as a janitor. Late at night I was invited to his home since it was too late to take a train to mine. At his house he noticed I was restless and offered a calming massage. This wasn't a particular fantasy of mine, and when he began to use different massage methods on my back, his hands slick with a geranium essential oil, I giggled because it tickled. Think of the movie *Dirty Dancing* when Patrick Swayze's character moved his hand up and down Baby's waist to arm. So, in the end, there was no massage but the sweet scent of geranium oil made a long-lasting good impression on me. And I did get shut-eye that evening.

1 ounce jojoba oil
1 ounce almond oil
5 drops jasmine essential oil
5 drops rose essential oil
5 drops geranium essential oil
5 drops orange essential oil
10 drops sandalwood essential oil

Make a base by mixing jojoba and almond oils. Set aside. Add the essential oils, and then combine with the base oils.

Later on, you'll discover not only can geranium be a go-to essential oil for massages, but its usage in blends for other things will make you feel at home wherever you are. Meanwhile, let's take a look at ginger—a beloved oil of mine, especially in food.

SCENT-SATIONAL HEALING OILS SHORT & SWEET

✓ Take note of geranium and its powers, especially for women, due to its linalool compound, for one, because we know it has a calming effect.
✓ Do realize the compound geraniol makes geranium essential oil act like nature's antidepressant without side effects such as weight gain and insomnia.
✓ This floral oil heals in a variety of ways with its eugenol, and like eucalyptus, it helps fight off inflammation to infections.
✓ Geranium has a multitude of uses and methods to apply it, from inhaling, topical, and consuming it, too . . . It is a go-to essential oil that is underrated and deserves more recognition.

Ginger

(Zingiber officinale)

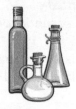

E's all 'ot and an' ginger when alive
An' 'e's generally shammin' when 'e's dead.
—RUDYARD KIPLING

Spicy ginger oil, not unlike geranium oil, enlivened my female passion as a shy teenager. In my mid-teens I still felt awkward with curly hair that frizzed in fog and rain. I was isolated and didn't connect with people until one summer. The charismatic boy next door gave me attention. He was older, handsome, magnetic like ginger oil, but engaged to be married.

One summer night, I paid him a visit. We sat on the front porch wooden swing and talked late into the night about dreams, life, and adventures we had yet to experience. I shared fresh gingerbread my mom had baked. The ginger oil she had used gave the cupcakes an earthy aroma and flavor that was enticing. We both nibbled on the moist cakes. The air was warm and humid; but I felt attractive complete with blushing, and connecting with a boy. It was the beginning of blossoming into a woman. I wondered for a long time after that evening of flirting under the Full Moon, "Can ginger oil be a love potion?"

THE ROOTS OF GINGER

It is believed gold, frankincense, and myrrh were the gifts brought by the three wise men from the east and ginger (rhizomes were used to extract essential oil) was the gift of the one Wiseman who didn't finish the journey to Bethlehem. His last days in Syria included giving ginger roots to a rabbi who cared for him, as he was sick. The rabbi told him a powerful king would come to be born in Bethlehem or the "House of Bread." The rabbi instructed his students to create houses of bread to nourish hope for their Messiah.

Historians will tell you that ginger was believed to be an aphrodisiac according to the Persian doctor Avicenna who mixed it with honey. This gave the blend a syrupy texture. It was used to enhance libido. A strong aroma—such as ginger essential oil with a warm scent—can enhance good feelings and boost circulation. Also, women in Senegal lure men by wearing ginger in their belts. So maybe that memorable night was due to the ginger after all.[1]

Ginger is not a new essential oil. The oil can be traced back to the beginning of time. As French legend goes, gingerbread was brought to Europe in 992 by an Armenian monk, later Saint Gregory Nicolas. He taught gingerbread cooking to purists and other Christians. Historians believe gingerbread (which could have been made with a homemade oil), was baked in Europe at the end of the tenth century. Gingerbread was popular in Germany during the fifteenth century, and Germany ended up being called the "Gingerbread Capital of the World." This, in turn, intrigued people and captivated interest and perpetuated the love of gingerbread to be enjoyed in the Mediterranean countries throughout Europe. Swedish nuns baked gingerbread to ease indigestion, while gingerbread biscuits shaped like important guests were served from Elizabeth I of England in her court.

GINGER ESSENTIALS

Ginger oil comes from the plant's stems and is extracted by way of steam and CO_2 distillation. This spicy oil contains many healing properties, including antioxidants, such as phytochemicals, polyphenols, tannins, and terpenes. More than one hundred powerful components have been found in gingerroot. Therapeutic benefits from ginger oil resin act as an antioxidant and an anti-inflammatory agent.

Also, made up of mostly sesquiterpenes, it's no surprise researchers show ginger essential oil may fight both bacterial-related health problems and inflammation. Also, gingerols and shogals are noted components in ginger and gets noticed for their potential healing powers for a variety of ailments.[2]

Other important components include zingiberene, b-sesquiphellandrene, and other compounds like ar-curcumen, B-bisabolene, linalool, and geranial. These properties help ginger essential oil aid in health ailments and have been noted in scientific studies.

MEDICINAL POWERS OF GINGER OIL

Research shows gingerroot is a digestive aid, like cinnamon, that can be soothing medicine for the stomach and intestines, relieving indigestion, cramps, and nausea. Studies prove that ginger in different forms, from capsules to tea, can help stave off the queasy feeling if you don't have your sea legs and/or must cope with choppy waters.

It's the gingerols and shogals in ginger essential oil that help keep motion sickness at bay, so to speak. How exactly does it do that? These two compounds help inhibit nausea by relaxing the smooth muscles in the stomach. Also, the parasympathetic nervous system can trigger salivary secretions with the help of ginger oil neutralizing acid in the stomach. That means, it may lessen that queasy feeling we all have experienced one time or another. We want to feel normal ASAP and if ginger oil can come to the rescue, why would you not give it a try?

What's more, the antioxidants and anti-inflammatory properties in ginger oil can help ease joint pain. Ginger oil should be mixed with a carrier oil. Light olive oil is my personal choice since it also fights inflammation and can reduce tenderness and swelling in aching muscles.

Additional Advantages: Ginger oil can lessen motion sickness, but it can also work for morning sickness during pregnancy, food poisoning, or queasiness from a medication. It's my go-to remedy if my stomach is acting up from a bout of the flu. I often will munch on gingersnaps or ginger tea made with hot water and 1 drop of essential oil.

Come On, Try It! Ginger oil can be used in blends for an aromatherapy massage. It is infused in soaps and gels for a shower or bath. It can be inhaled from the bottle, candles, and incense. It can also be used on small pads and put into aromatic jewelry. Ginger oil is a popular culinary oil that can be enjoyed in savory and sweet dishes to add a warming, spicy flavor and with a rich aroma.

Comforting Gingerbread Squares with Lemon Oil Frosting

❖ ❖ ❖

When I was introduced to the world of sailing, it was an adventure that I was hesitant about. I passed on the voyage to Benicia, Northern California, with a mate (who took one sailing class) maneuvering through the choppy waters. I drove and met him at the boat, which I did sleep on. I munched on gingersnaps at night because the water moved the twenty-seven-foot vessel back and forth. I like being on the water, but sometimes motion sickness can be difficult on my stomach. Munching on gingersnaps or sipping ginger tea takes the edge off. This recipe is better than using a gingerbread store-bought mix. It's flavorful, moist, and with a drop of ginger oil and lemon oil you get a wave of taste to write home about.

CAKE

¾ dark brown sugar
¾ cup molasses
½ cup European-style butter (1 stick), melted (save a
    tablespoon for greasing baking dish)
2 organic brown eggs
2½ cups all-purpose flour
2 teaspoons baking soda
1 teaspoon cinnamon
½ teaspoon allspice
1 cup hot water
1 drop ginger essential oil
2 teaspoons lemon rind
½ cup crystallized ginger pieces

In a large mixing bowl, combine sugar, molasses, butter, and eggs. Stir until smooth. Set aside. In a medium-size bowl, mix flour, baking soda, cinnamon, and allspice. Combine sugar, molasses, butter, and egg mixture to dry ingredients. Add water. Mix thoroughly. Stir in essential oil. Fold in lemon rind and ginger pieces. Use an 8-inch by 8-inch baking dish (grease with oil or butter). Pour batter into it. Bake at 350 degrees F for about 40 minutes or until the top is firm. Do not overbake. Cool.

Makes about 10 squares.

LEMON OIL FROSTING

1 cup confectioners sugar
3 tablespoons organic 2 percent low-fat milk
1 drop lemon essential oil
1 teaspoon honey
½ teaspoon pure vanilla extract
Whipped cream (optional)
Mint sprigs (optional)

In a mixing bowl, combine sugar, milk, oil, honey, and extract. Stir well or blend with a mixer until smooth and creamy. Frost gingerbread squares piped with lemon oil frosting. Serve square with a dollop of whipped cream topped with mint sprigs.

It's time to put the ginger oil back in the kitchen pantry and bring out another healing oil to sniff and fall in love with. In the next chapter, I'll praise an oil that is derived from flowers and contains many healing compounds, just like ginger.

SCENT-SATIONAL HEALING OILS SHORT & SWEET

✓ Remember, ginger essential oil contains hydrocarbons like sesquiterpenes, which can help lessen bacterial infections and inflammation.

✓ It's the gingerols and shogals in ginger essential oil that relax the stomach and fight motion sickness on the sea, car, or in the air.

✓ Antioxidant-rich ginger oil with its health and culinary uses is recognized around the world as a healing medicine.

✓ Do note, ginger is a versatile culinary spicy oil, like clove and nutmeg, which can add flavor to nutrient-dense savory and sweet dishes year-round.

✓ Don't ignore the aphrodisiac folklore and real anecdotal positive effects of ginger oil for both women and men. If it works to boost your libido despite what wary scientists say, carry on and reap the benefits of this spicy essential oil. ·

Jasmine

(*Jasminum officinalis* and *J. grandiflorum*)

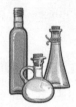

Jasmine, the name of which signifies fragrance,
is the emblem of delicacy and elegance.
—DORTHEA DIX

The word "jasmine" takes me back to fun nights and an adventure-loving gal-pal, a Montessori teacher from Taiwan. She named her school after jasmine, the sensual flower. In hindsight, I recall she wore the essential oil from Taiwan every time we went club hopping in San Francisco. Her goal was to meet a man and get married—and jasmine was her "bait" she told me. And that essential oil tool confession spawned a flashback to my college days . . .

In my late teens, I was a student at West Valley Junior College in Saratoga, California. My best gal pal and I were physical education majors, which led to physical activity. Many times we rode our ten-speed bicycles for hours. One night it was our goal to make it to San

Jose State University, a place known for its all-night parties. Thanks to bike riding I was energized and feeling confident. Before we left on our adventure into the night, she shared her cologne, a blend with an exotic-smelling jasmine essential oil, which I put on my wrists.

To this day I believe it was the scent of this magical potion that led to a magical evening. I drew a lot of attention from the students in the fraternity house. We played the game Truth or Dare and with my nickname "gutsy," I reaped the reward of meeting someone special. Aromatherapists claim jasmine has aphrodisiac qualities, and in hindsight I will not disagree that the power of jasmine—a sweet and floral fragrance—played a part in my new romance, a lasting summer love..

THE ROOTS OF JASMINE

Jasmine essential oil has Asian roots, but aromatherapists will tell you the best quality comes from France and Italy. Jasmine, coined "queen of the night" in India, was used as an aphrodisiac and may have enhanced spiritual growth. For centuries, women have used perfumes and cosmetics made with jasmine. It is believed that the sweet smelling and striking jasmine flower is a sign of happiness and true love.

The scent of jasmine flowers has also been linked with love and romance from the past during "First Nights" in Asian countries. Aromatherapists share the antics of the bride and groom who allegedly infused their room with the flowery scent to lessen performance anxiety, and the benefits resulted in less inhibitions and more romantic feelings.

A Love Connection with Jasmine

Lynda Ballard of the United Kingdom–based Kobashi Ltd. essential oils company, recalls a memorable experience with jasmine. See how, in her own words, this floral oil was a gift to cherish . . .

I had put a dab of pure jasmine oil, renowned for its exotic and sensual properties, on my pulse points. I met Scott while selling Kobashi essential oils at a "Mind, Body, Spirit" fair in 1994. It was in the town of Totnes in Devon. He came by my stand and commented on the wonderful aroma. I told him, "It is jasmine." He asked if he could have my phone number. I gave him Kobashi's number. We have been married now for nearly twenty-five years. He still loves jasmine. Scott adds, "I love Lynda more than jasmine." He adds, "Jasmine was there to help break the ice."

JASMINE ESSENTIALS

No surprise that jasmine oil comes from the flowers, and is CO_2 solvent-extracted into a rich and expensive absolute. Jasmine essential oil contains about one hundred chemical properties—not just one. The primary healing compounds include benzyl acetate and benzyl benzoate—which have antibacterial and antiviral powers. Other components include the calming medicinal compound linalool (no wonder I was uninhibited at the fraternity) and geraniol.

But this super essential oil also is touted for its calming benefits, not unlike chamomile oil. Its chill effect is due to a neurotransmitter or brain chemical (famma-aminobutyric acid) that can help reduce anxiety.

MEDICINAL POWERS OF JASMINE OIL

Because of its antiviral compounds it also can lower the risk of developing respiratory infections, too. Jasmine essential oil can ease nervous system disorders, including anxiety, stress, and insomnia, which can wreak havoc on the immune system. Past studies show this powerful oil can slow breathing, lower heart rate, and help you to feel calmer. And if you are destressed and get adequate sleep, it will bolster your immune system.

Researchers report in the *Journal of Biological Chemistry* that the scent of jasmine can trigger the GABA response, which is a chemical messenger that travels through the brain and nervous system inhibiting nerve cells and controls anxiety. This, in turn, means inhaling the essential oil from a vial or in a massage can make you feel relaxed—like popping a valium but without the side effects of a prescription drug. Here's proof: Hundreds of fragrances were tested in both humans and lab rats to find out their effect on GABA receptors. It was discovered that floral jasmine boosted the GABA effect, acting like a sedative. The lead scientist in the study, Professor Hanns Hett, believes the benefits of jasmine validate scientific evidence, backing up that aromatherapy can work to aid in health.[1]

Additional Advantages: The flowery fragrant jasmine essential oil is used on wounds to help prevent infection. What's more, since jasmine essential oil can calm the nervous system, it can enhance lovemaking as noted with historical Asian honeymooners. And today, sex has many healing virtues, including strengthening the immune system, burning calories, lessening pain, and enhancing better sleep—all can lead to better health and living longer, richer lives.

Come On, Try It! A mutual jasmine oil massage or burning a jasmine candle can not only be calming but it can boost mood and increase energy. It's often inhaled or applied to the skin. Aromatherapists recommend aromatic massage using jasmine oil with lotions and carrier oils, too.[2] It is also used in cosmetics, incense, and perfume.

Mood Boosting Jasmine Perfume

I am more of a woodsy essential oil scent fan when it comes to perfume but on occasion a floral fragrance is a pleasing change. Often, it uplifts my spirits when I wear it. As a teen in the early sixties, I wore White Shoulders, which was a soft white-floral cologne. It was a popular inexpensive perfume with a floral-woodsy blend, including rose, sandalwood, musk, and jasmine. One Valentine's Day, my dad gave me a gold heart photo locket with flower etchings on it. Nowadays, I insert a pad with a drop of jasmine oil in it and put the charm on a bracelet. The floral scent triggers memories of my late father who left me a jasmine and cat watercolor painting. When traveling I wear it to make me feel protected. It is a link to my father who has my heart eternally. This recipe for a homemade perfume is inspired by my childhood, and my father, who introduced me to the limitless world of aromatic flowers and plants.

2 drops jasmine absolute (An absolute is like the essential oil, extracted from jasmine flowers but has a stronger aroma, is more concentrated, and costly.)
12 drops rose essential oil
3 drops neroli essential oil
3 drops sandalwood essential oil
1 ounce jojoba oil

Swirl together the jasmine absolute and the essential oils. Add to the jojoba oil. Apply this classic, floral scent on the neck, between the breasts, or inside the elbows.

Now that you have added another essential oil to your must-have collection, let's move on to the next essential oil—my favorite. Living in the Golden State—I have discovered there are lavender farms in the central and southern regions—what I shared with you in chapter 1 wasn't all a pipe dream.

SCENT-SATIONAL HEALING OILS SHORT & SWEET

✓ Jasmine oil has many virtues, such as aiding in better sleep, lessening pain, and boosting self-esteem and confidence, which helps enhance well-being.
✓ One of jasmine's most celebrated benefits is that it's nature's sedative due to its GABA calming compound, which affects the brain in a positive way.
✓ Combining floral jasmine oil with earthy and citrus essential oils provides a nice balance and a plethora of healing powers . . .
✓ Not only is it a pleasurable fragrance to wear jasmine, essential oil can be a used in a destressing aromatic massage or bath.

Lavender

(*Lavandula angustifolia*)

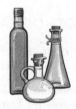

Hot lavender, mints, savory, marjoram.
The marigold, that goes to bed with the sun and him rise
weeping.
—William Shakespeare, *The Winter's Tale*

During my on-the-road travels, Eugene, Oregon, was a place I stopped and lived for a short span. I recall housesitting for a down-to-earth couple. The woman, a natural hippie who could chop wood and cite the healing powers of teas and essential oils, introduced me to homemade lavender essential oil.

The small cabin did not have a bathtub. At this time in my life, while I was raised in a comfortable Mediterranean climate, I wasn't used to a lot of rain or cold temperatures. I faltered igniting and using the woodstove. To warm up, I escaped to the shower. Sitting down on the stall floor, I bathed in a homemade DIY lavender body wash. Once through, I was relaxed and went to bed early. That night, due to the cold air where I could see my breath, I cuddled up with my black Lab Stonefox who provided warmth. At midnight, I woke up.

I felt the small house was warmer; the stove did heat up (perhaps an ember was to thank). The banana nut–lavender bread batter (I used the homemade lavender oil) I had stored in the fridge was ready to bake! One hour later: it was baked bread. I let it cool on the countertop, and covered it with a cloth like a child in bed. I slept through the cold winter's night and awoke to a sweet and floral-scented lavender bread slice with a cup of hot tea at dawn.

THE ROOTS OF LAVENDER

Welcome to the word "lavender" which comes from the Latin word *"lavera,"* meaning "to wash." After all, the Romans used lavender in their baths to reduce fatigue and loosen up painful joints.

Actually, for more than twenty-five hundred years medicinal uses of lavender have been noted in history. The earliest record may be Egypt for its usage in mummification. Its versatility, from therapeutic uses to religious ceremonies, was enjoyed in a variety of cultures. The Romans loved lavender for its aromatherapy benefits, and cooking.

Medieval Europeans believed it to be an aphrodisiac and calming. And for centuries, the healing aroma of lavender flowers were used to help sick people in hospitals and homes to recover.

LAVENDER ESSENTIALS

Lavender oil comes from the flower. The oil is extracted by steam and CO_2 distillation from the flowering tops. Lavender has different species, including spike lavender. The primary workhorses of lavender essential oil are its antioxidants, which make it one of the leaders of the pack among other oils providing it with a multitude of health benefits. It is one of the most popular essential oils although it's not a prescribed medicine.

Lavender contains dozens and dozens of healing compounds. The main properties reported in the *Journal of Chromatography* include acetate, monoterpeneoids and sesquiteerpenoids, linalool and linalyl acetate, ocimene, also some lavandulyl acetate, terpinen-4-ol and lavandulol, and camphor.[1]

MEDICINAL POWERS OF LAVENDER OIL

Researchers believe it's the antioxidant disease fighters that may help protect against neurological disorders, work against infections from bacteria, and aid in metabolic issues, from diabetes to liver and kidney problems.

Stacks of studies show that lavender essential oil is one of the top contenders in the world of essential oils. It's touted for easing one big problem that plagues the nation—stress. We live in a time when feeling on edge happens due to pressures from work, family, finances, and experiencing love and loss. However, turning to natural alternatives like calming lavender essential oil may be helpful as an aid to help provide a sense of calm and normalcy so we can cope better with challenges.

There have been countless studies on the benefits of lavender to help treat anxiety, depression, and insomnia, which can overlap in the twenty-first century. Research has been conducted on lab rodents and humans (like the mouse and man Charley in the bittersweet novel *Flowers for Algernon*). In some studies, an oral lavender oil pill (Silexan) was taken by people and within weeks showed positive results. Also, small clinical studies have shown lavender oil aromatherapy can help lessen anxiety. It is believed by scientists that lavender may trigger the feel-good brain chemical serotonin that can make you feel happier.[2]

Lavender is an essential oil that is touted for its antiseptic, antiviral and antibacterial properties, which can help treat respiratory infections, lessen inflammation—the culprit of many chronic and acute health conditions—and soothe aches and pains in the joints and muscles. Speaking of muscles... I recall a dentist who told me he used lavender oil in his office. The essential oil in a diffuser worked to help calm his patients.

Meet an Essential Aromatherapist Extraordinaire

Enter Retha Nesmith, Certified Aromatherapist of Plant Therapy in Twin Fall, Idaho. She grew up using essential oils, thanks to her mom, so healing oils were part of her roots. In 2012 she began working for Plant Therapy, a blossoming essential oil company. After fielding questions from inquisitive customers, Retha thought it would be beneficial to obtain a certificate in aromatherapy—and she did just that, giving credit to Aromahead Institute. Since then, the kid who remembered the smell of tea tree oil in her childhood has grown up into an adult who is an essential oils advocate. Her mission is to help people on their journey in the land of essential oils and aromatherapy. In an exclusive interview, I asked the aromatherapist about her own interest in essential oils and how she uses them in home remedies and to promote well-being.

Q: *What are your favorite oils?*

A: Lavender is such a versatile essential oil, I use it in many different ways. Mostly, I use it for skin concerns, such as a bee sting or dry skin. I also like to diffuse lemon oil with peppermint to give me a boost of energy. Peppermint is great during the summer months to help cool me off. I also use it for headaches and to help with an energy boost. And then Vetiver . . .

Q: *Did you fall in love with one essential oil?*

A: I absolutely love Vetiver and I know that Vetiver is often a scent that people do not like. Every time I smell Vetiver my body is overcome by relaxation. My muscles loosen up, my eyes close. I can feel my body breathing. It is really an amazing thing! And every time this happens, I think to myself, How could anybody not love this scent? When I am too stressed, tired, or just overwhelmed, I go to Vetiver— a definite in my house.

Q: *Do you personally use edible essential oils?*

A: I do a little bit. I have used some essential oils in cooking. I also use essential oils internally for medicinal purpose on a rare occasion.

Q: *Share an unforgettable aromatherapy experience at home or on a getaway.*

A: I don't have one single oil that is my favorite for massage or tub time. However, my favorite blend of essential oils contains frankincense fereana, bergamot, and lavender. Honestly, I am not a huge fan of the scent lavender, but lavender combined with the bright aroma bergamot and the sweet but grounding scent of frankincense fereana is heavenly. The first time I smelled this blend it instantly relaxed me and I knew it was going to be a favorite of mine, and now I use it in my bubble baths.

Q: *If you were whisked away to an isolated cabin vacay and could only use three essential oils—what are they and what would you use them for?*

A: Lavender is my go-to for sunburns (if I'm in a cabin for a weekend I better be enjoying the fresh air outside). Lavender is also great for so many skin issues such as bug bites. Whenever I spend time outdoors, I always make sure I have lavender on me. Vetiver is my go-to oil for relaxation and focus. Weekend getaways can be stressful. You aren't in your own bed; your mind is often wandering because of all the work you could be getting done. I enjoy adding Vetiver to a personal inhaler or simply inhaling it right out of the bottle. It instantly calms my mind, and my whole body feels relaxed and ready to take on whatever comes my way!

Additional Advantages: Versatile lavender, from purple fields in a Mediterranean climate, is an all-purpose essential oil for minor health ailments, too. And it is a known comforting oil since its compounds can calm down brain waves and reduce stress. Also, you can savor lavender-chamomile essential oil in beverages, like tea, which acts as a sedative due to its component linalool; this, in turn, can have a relaxing effect on the nervous system. Lavender oil can also be used to help heal scars, lessen stretch marks, and soothe insect bites. (Refer to part 4, "Home Remedies.")

Come On, Try It! Lavender oil is infused in beauty and cleaning products. Inhaling this oil in a steaming vaporizer or putting a drop or two on a cotton ball is a sure-fire way to chill. It can be used undiluted and massaged on body parts, like when I twisted my ankle after allowing my dog to walk me. People, including me, do use lavender in a variety of methods, from aromatherapy candles, baths, to spa massages, home cures—even in foods. When used in cooking and baking, lavender oil is added in muffins, cakes, frosting, tea blends, and even ice cream. Ah, the lavender essential oil is a well-loved natural wonder and deserves adoration.

Invigorating
Lavender's Lovely DIY Olive Oil Balm

❖ ❖ ❖

One winter a magazine editor sent a professional photographer to my home for a photo shoot. I didn't wear a lot of makeup for my photos, but I did wear a clear lip gloss, eye liner, mascara—and a lavender-scented essential body oil perfume, which calmed me. I felt and looked relaxed in the photos, posing with my Brittany spaniel, since a dog was part of the story. These days, I've learned you can make your own lip balm and it's custom-tailored to the essential oil of your choice—including lavender.

The North American Olive Oil Association believes your friends and family will love this DIY olive oil balm. Made with all-natural ingredients including extra virgin olive oil, this olive oil balm can be used for lips, hands, or anything that needs care this winter. This lip balm with lavender is inspired by that special day that provides memories of my beloved canine.

1 cup extra virgin olive oil
2 ounces beeswax pastilles (you can substitute camellia or carnauba wax)
1 teaspoon vitamin E oil
Essential oil of your choice such as bergamot, ylang-ylang, lavender, sage, or rose
Tins or jars to hold the balm

STOVETOP DIRECTIONS

Set up a double boiler to melt the wax with indirect heat. Put the beeswax and olive oil into the double-boiler. Stir until the wax is melted. When melted, stir in the vitamin E oil. While still liquid, pour the balm into tins or small mason jars. Stir in 10–20 drops of essential oil (depending on how strong the scent should be). Leave overnight to solidify.

MICROWAVE DIRECTIONS

You can also use a microwave to make the olive oil balm. Use a glass, wide mouth bowl, or mason jar. Do not use a plastic container. Put the beeswax and olive oil into the glass container and microwave for 30 or 40 seconds. Stir and repeat until the mixture is liquid. When melted, stir in the vitamin E oil. While still liquid, pour the balm into tins or small mason jars. Stir in 10–20 drops of essential oil, depending on how strong the scent should be. Leave overnight to solidify.

To clean up, wipe the mixture while still liquid, re-heating your containers if necessary. Small amounts of wax residue can be washed out normally using dish soap and a sponge. Do not let large amounts of the wax mixture go down the drain, as it will cool and solidify and possibly cause clogged drains!

(Courtesy: North American Olive Oil Association)

Take a break with a lavender blend bath or aromatic massage. Get ready. It's time to give the next refreshing essential oil a chance to win you over. I'll show you why versatile lemon essential oil is an all-time favorite.

SCENT-SATIONAL HEALING OILS SHORT & SWEET

✓ Do you have a cut, blemish, bite, or puncture? Lavender essential oil is a super skin care remedy to help heal inflammation and soothe the redness, swelling, and help speed up the recovery process which may be due to the compounds monoterpenoids and sesquiteerpenoids.

✓ Lavender essential oil is calming due to the compound linalool that can help you to destress . . .

✓ And note, if you are calm you are lowering your risk of developing high blood pressure, heart disease, and possibly cancer.

✓ Don't forget that pairing lavender with other essential oils works well.

Lemon

(Citrus limon)

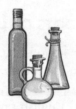

Know'st the land where the lemon trees bloom,
Where the gold orange glows in the deep thickets
   gloom
Where a wind ever soft from the blue heaven blows,
And the groves are of laurel and myrtle and rose.
     —JOHANN VON GOETHE

After a short and cold, bittersweet escapade in Oregon, with memories of lavender oil lingering in my mind, I came back to California, my home. I reentered college as a grad student. After a day and night of classes, I'd bypass my apartment and go to the gym for rest and rejuvenation. One night the spa offered a complimentary essential oil aromatic massage. I hesitated to partake in the service not knowing what to expect. But I did it. A sophisticated, older European spa tech with a Swedish accent was my masseuse. He used a citrus lemon essential oil fragrance as the base mixed with a sweet almond oil. His massage techniques worked their magic as I felt my muscles loosen up, and nervous tension vanished as my cluttered mind cleared like deleting typewritten words on a page.

Once home-based, I was greeted by my loyal Labrador, Stonefox. It was like the grueling day full of back-to-back classes, tests, and home-work didn't happen. My sensitive canine seemed calmer thanks to my vibe. To this day, I credit the fresh scent of lemon oil that gave me back a sense of balance.

THE ROOTS OF LEMON

Lemon oil comes from the lemon tree, which has roots in Asia, but has been linked to Italy since the fourth century. Food historians and aromatherapists believe Europeans used lemons to fight contagious illnesses such as malaria, and English sailors used lemons as a scurvy remedy to protect against a lack of an adequate amount of vitamin C.

Citrus oils, like lemon, are fresh and light with an invigorating fra-grance—used in ancient times to perfume clothes and keep away pesky bugs, like flies and creepy-crawlies. In the twentieth century, I recall my mom would use fresh lemon juice and water to clean appli-ances in the kitchen, giving the air a refreshing scent. But its magical components can do so much more.

LEMON ESSENTIALS

Extracted by cold-pressing the citrus peel, the key compound in lemon essential oil that scientists have identified is d-limonene. It may be the property that makes this popular and versatile oil so in-credibly powerful to fight infection and disease. What's more, re-search shows lemon oil has cancer-fighting power.

Other healing compounds in this citrus essential oil are alcohols, aldehydes, esters, sesquiterpenes, sterols, and terpenes—all con-tribute to lemon oil's wide variety of therapeutic powers. To be more concise, the breakdown of properties in lemon oil include a-pinene, camphene, b-pinene, sabinene, myrcene, a-terpinene, linalool, and b-bisobolene.

Naturally, the antioxidants such as flavonoids (powerful disease fighters) in lemon essential oil likely play a role in making this citrus oil a health-giving wonder, too. This citrus essential oil comes with anti-inflammatory and antimicrobial properties, which are helpful for many ailments.

MEDICINAL POWERS OF LEMON OIL

Research proves that lemon essential oil can and does come to the rescue with restorative and recovery benefits. German scientists show that d-limonene, which is found in its citrusy cousins, may slow down tumors from growing and boost what's called "apoptosis"—a cancer fighter.[1]

Healing lemon essential oil with its mighty flavonoids may also help to fight allergies, carcinogens, inflammation, and viruses. These super antioxidants may also lower the "bad" LDL cholesterol, which may lower your risk of heart disease and stroke.

And the fresh and exhilarating fragrance—think of fresh-squeezed lemon juice in a glass of iced cold lemonade on a hot summer day—may help to stave off depression.

Essential lemon oil has a multitude of uses from a healthful massage, like I enjoyed, to being a healing oil for ailments and protector against specific diseases. It is touted, though, for its medicinal qualities around the globe. Yes, this citrus oil can be used to relieve coughs, fevers, and a sore throat. Ever use fresh lemon slices in a cup of hot tea when you have a cold or flu? There's a reason behind that home remedy!

Additional Advantages: The healing powers of essential lemon oil don't stop there. It can also help boost physical and mental energy, quell nausea, relieve a cough and sore throat, detoxify your body, and even help in weight loss. (You can find out more in the chapter "The Slimming Essentials.")

Research shows that antibacterial lemon essential oil is one of the most potent healing oils, especially when it comes to fighting bacteria, including germs we hear about people getting from touching infected surfaces like on an airplane, workplace, or grocery store—even at home from our family members who may have touched infected surfaces with germs. Speaking of home, you can make your own lemon fresh soap to stay germ-free.

Come On, Try It! Lemon essential oil and aromatherapy are used in beauty products, soaps, and household cleaners. Its light scent is believed to pick up your spirits, and disinfect you from bacteria whether you're using a body wash or washing dishes. Lemon oil can be inhaled from a vial or diffuser. It also can be diluted and used with carrier oils for massages and baths. It also is a popular culinary oil used in cooking and baking as well as used in a water beverage.

Bacterial Fighting
Citrus Liquid Hand Soap

If you don't want to use store-bought hand soap, this DIY method is not difficult. The best part is not only will it be nature's best, you can benefit from a variety of citrusy fragrances. Here is a liquid hand soap recipe. It contains germ-fighting citrus essential oils, and knowing this will give you peace of mind when you wash your hands, especially during flu and cold season.

1 cup castile soap
2 tablespoons sweet almond essential oil
2 teaspoons vitamin E oil
50 drops sweet orange essential oil
50 drops steam distilled lemon essential oil
30 drops steam distilled essential lime

Mix all ingredients in a pump bottle. Store in a cool place. Use as needed.

(Courtesy: Plant Therapy)

Now you'll be more enthusiastic to name lemon essential oil as your must-have oil, but let's not ignore other favorites to come! I'll show you how the next essential oil, much like lemon since it is citrusy, doesn't get the praise it deserves. Lemon oil is popular but this lesser known counterpart is one that you should become familiar with and add to your oil repertoire.

SCENT-SATIONAL HEALING OILS SHORT & SWEET

✓ Stay aware of how lemon essential oil can help you to fight off infectious diseases because of its powerful antimicrobial compounds, including d-limonene, sesquiterpenes, and terpenes, and to help strengthen your immune system.
✓ And note, the antioxidants such as flavonoids (powerful disease fighters) in citrus essential oils provide anti-inflammatory properties.
✓ Not only can this citrus oil guard your body from respiratory infections thanks to its antioxidants, it can recharge the mind and spirit.
✓ Since scientists admit they aren't yet able to say essential oils can cure cancer, you can use the compound d-limonene-rich lemon oil, which may inhibit tumors from growing . . . this could be used by elderly men who have stage 1 prostate cancer that has not metastasized.
✓ Know that citrus essential oils, like lemon infused in an antibacterial soap, can be a super germ-fighting potion during flu and cold season.

Orange

(Citrus sinensis)

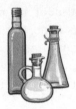

Did you ever sleep in a field of orange-trees in
* bloom?*
The air which one inhales deliciously is quin-
* tessence of perfumes.*

          —GUY DE MAUPASSANT

Orange is another citrus oil scent that has made its imprint on my body and spirit, as it may do for you, too. Its lively aroma is fresh and vibrant and can be calming and invigorating. Orange essential oil has befriended me, especially one unforgettable time.

When I took a semester off from college due to financial chaos, I was hired by a European man to clean a large estate owned by his grandparents. In need of housing, I was put in the back cottage—which was lacking a shower or bathtub. The man's grandmother didn't speak English, but her actions spoke loud and clear: She didn't like me—an interloper. I was another woman inside her cluttered kitchen. It was my job to clean. After a week of hard work amid hostile vibes, the woman made a deal with me. I could take a bath if I would vacate the premises.

The Victorian home boasted a large, claw-foot bathtub, oversized fluffy towels, and an array of old-world bath oils—including a dusty vial with the word "orange." I ran the hot water and the steam paired with the scent of fresh oranges. I escaped into a relaxing utopia of a bath. The steam filled the air, reminding me of the San Francisco fog. I transcended into another place for about thirty minutes. But it was that quality time that uplifted my spirits and gave me the courage to get dressed, grab my knapsack and canine, and move on to an oasis—a shoebox-size studio with a hot plate—situated on the San Francisco Bay Area peninsula in the middle of nowhere. And it is the citrus scent both sedating and invigorating of orange essential oil that often takes me back to this solo spiritual journey of being strong.

THE ROOTS OF ORANGE

Aromatherapists trace orange essential oil back to the biblical times because citrus was prevalent and used for food and survival. Throughout centuries, oranges were eaten by cultures around the globe. Orange trees were introduced to the Mediterranean countries by the Saracens during the Crusades. It is found in Italy, Israel, Spain, and in the United States, including my home state, California. The essential oil provides different varieties of orange oils such as neroli or orange blossom essential oil, and blood orange essential oil, which depends on its roots (yes, literally).

ORANGE ESSENTIALS

Orange, sometimes called orange sweet oil, is cold-pressed from the peel, like lemon oil, and also contains the component d-limonene, which is a major compound in this oil. Limonene is an anti-cancer compound, because it may help slow down tumor growth in cancer due to the changes it creates in cells, according to past research.

Other healing properties, like phytochemicals, may halt the growth of cancer, especially lung cancer, as reported by Chinese researchers in the *Molecular Nutrition Food Research* journal. More research is needed before orange essential oil is accepted as a cancer fighter in the world of science, but it's not to be ignored.[1]

Other compounds in orange essential oil include a-pinene, myrcene, sabinene, linalool, citronellol, and geranial. There are many different kinds of orange oil, including bitter orange, blood orange, neroli, sweet orange, and tangerine, which includes the same compounds of its counterpart. And, of course, bergamot is an essential oil that I have used in body care blends.

Bergamot—A Heart-Healthy Hybrid of Orange Oil

I have utilized bergamot (*Citrus bergamia*) in multiple ways from candles to Earl Grey tea. Originally from Asia, the fruit bergamot grows in Italy present-day; bergamot oil caught my attention because of its healing virtues. There are multiple past studies showing bergamot in the workplace can help lower heart rate and blood pressure in employees.

In one Taiwan study, fifty-four elementary school teachers were evaluated to see whether or not aroma could cause stress reduction. Bergamot essential oil was used as an aromatherapy spray for ten minutes. The results: a reduction in heart rate, which shows the oil affected the nervous system in a positive way and appears to drive the automatic nervous activity toward a balanced state.[2]

Other past medical research suggests the flavonoids, including alpha-pinene and limonene, may help relaxation, soothe anxiety, and lower stress levels. While I have de-stressing citrus oil on the table, here is a beverage for you.

Essential Citrus Julius

During the summertime I fall into a smoothie-fest. Citrus-flavored drinks spawn memories of the classic orange smoothie and frothy Orange Julius that I used to buy at malls—both indoor and outdoor. I learned how to whip up my own version of the orange smoothie, a sweet and natural drink created in the 1920s by Julius Freed. This recipe is inspired by the orange drinks I savored throughout the years. Adding citrus essential oils gives a flavorful spin on the blended beverage, adding a sweet and tart kick.

½ cup fresh orange juice
½ cup organic 2 percent low-fat milk or organic half-and-half
¾ cup all-natural premium French vanilla ice cream
2 tablespoons confectioners sugar
1 tablespoon honey
½ teaspoon pure vanilla extract
1 drop bergamot essential oil
1 drop blood orange essential oil
8–10 ice cubes
Fresh mint and orange slices for garnish

In a blender, combine juice, milk, and ice cream. Blend. Add sugar, honey, vanilla, and citrus essential oils. Add ice cubes, one by one, until smooth but thick. Add a bit more ice cream if you like it a creamier consistency. Pour in a parfait or milk shake glass. Add mint and orange slices on top, a straw and spoon.

Serves 1.

Medicinal Powers of Orange Oil

Unlike lemon oil, orange oil may be less antiseptic. However, it still merits healing powers especially for strengthening the immune system, which can help fight off colds and flu—possibly life-threatening for immune-compromised people, the very young, and elderly.

Studies show not only can orange oil lower anxiety, which is often linked to stress, but it can lower high blood pressure, too. And these intriguing findings about citrusy oil, like orange, show this essential oil may even help lower the risk of developing heart disease. The orange oil healing powers can help the mind. Here's proof.

The aromatherapy of citrus oils, including lemon and orange oils, may enhance brainpower. As people are living longer during the graying of America, an awareness of memory loss has grown substantially. This has affected dear friends in my life, who no longer remember me. It's a wake-up call, showing me how challenging cognitive decline can be for humans.

One study published in the journal *Psychogeriatrics* monitored twenty-eight elderly people coping with the scourge of dementia and/or Alzheimer's disease. The folks inhaled lemon and rosemary aromas in the morning followed by lavender and orange at night. The findings: There was an improvement in mental awareness of surroundings without ill side effects.[3]

Additional Advantages: This mood- and mind-enhancing essential oil can provide you with vigor and boundless vitality. Its antioxidant-rich properties can help fight colds and the flu. Orange essential oil also helps indigestion or queasiness. (Refer to part 4, "Home Remedies.") The fragrance of orange essential oil also may lower blood pressure and anxiety. This needs more research, but if it works for you, like it does for me, why wait?

Come On, Try It! Orange oil can be combined with other types of essential oils and used by inhalation methods with a vaporizer. It is also used in aromatic massages, baths, beauty soaps and shampoos, and even cleaning products. This fresh and fragrant citrus oil can be used in cooking and baking, too.

Essential Safety Tip: Citrus oils are to be used with caution and proper amounts, because they can be potent and cause irritation if you have sensitive skin. Do use with a carrier oil such as olive oil for topical use and in cooking and baking

Immunity Boosting
Orange Chocolate Bark

❖ ❖ ❖

During autumn I savor the colors of the leaves, the aroma of crisp air, and a crackling fire in the rock fireplace, and most of all fresh scented orange oil candles in the kitchen. One Thanksgiving in the Sierras I didn't follow in my mom's footsteps, which would have been getting up early in the morning to groom a twenty-pound turkey, making dressing from scratch, creating appetizers to put Martha Stewart to shame, and baking two pies. Instead, I took the Mediterranean route. I whipped up a batch of fall-style chocolate bark and brewed a pot of tea. I added orange essential oil into the white chocolate for a burst of citrus flavor. Since it wasn't heated long, I most likely got a dose of good-for-you antioxidants, which are also found in dark chocolate and nuts. This recipe is inspired by my love of fall. It has an essential oil no-cook twist, which will help change up your holidays and allow you to take a less hectic route if you decide to save a turkey and go rogue.

½ cup white chocolate chips or a bar (Ghirardelli)
½ cup dark chocolate chips or a bar (Ghirardelli)
½ teaspoon pure vanilla extract
1 drop orange essential oil
¼ cup each dried cranberries, glazed dried orange
    peel, raisins, chopped
¼ cup almonds, pecans, or walnuts, chopped

Melt dark chocolate in a microwave for about 1 minute. Place a paper towel over the bowl and keep an eye on it. Take the bowl out, stir, put back until smooth. Do not overcook. Add extract and essential oil, and mix well. Spread scented citrusy chocolate on a nonstick flat cookie sheet (or line with parchment paper). Spread and shape into a rectangle. Chill in freezer for about 10 minutes.

Meanwhile, melt white chocolate in the microwave. Once the chocolate is melted remove. Take out dark chocolate from the freezer and frost it with the white chocolate. Sprinkle with dried fruit mixture. Top with nuts. Refrigerate for about 20 minutes or until firm. Take out and place on a cutting board. Break into peanut brittle–size pieces for a nice rustic look. Place pieces into a plastic container. It stores nicely in the refrigerator or freezer.

Makes about 12 to 16 small pieces.

This quick and easy superfoods chocolate treat with an orange aroma is a sweet way to celebrate the season. Pair a piece or two with a cup of chamomile or lavender tea (use the leaves or bag—not an essential oil). Not only will this festive bark please your taste and smell, you'll feel energized by both!

Now that orange oil has made its way into your citrus essential oil collection, it's time to head back into the woods. I cherish the next oil more than life itself. Not only does it take me back in time to pleasant days and nights, having it on hand gives me a link to the past forever. Take a look at why the patchouli is an ancient essential oil that may stoke memories for you, too.

SCENT-SATIONAL HEALING OILS SHORT & SWEET

✓ Using orange oil with its antimicrobial properties, such as phyto-chemicals, can help keep germs at bay when used as a disinfec-tant, topically, inhaled, or ingested.

✓ Orange, like lemon essential oil, contains d-limonene, which is believed to be an anti-cancer compound, because it may help slow down tumor growth in cancer.

✓ Do realize heart-healthy healing compounds are found in berg-amot, an essential oil linked to orange oil, with its flavonoids that can help you to destress and lower anxiety levels.

✓ You can increase alertness by using orange essential oil. Research shows mental awareness of surroundings is possible by inhaling the citrus oil.

✓ Orange oil is a popular culinary oil used in cooking and baking that provides antioxidants. It is a healthful immune-enhancing oil to use in water, tea, and food. (Refer to chapter 29 for recipes that use orange essential oil in salad dressings, entrées, and desserts.)

✓ And notice, orange essential oil because of its bacteria-fighting antioxidants is used in cleaning products (refer to the healthy household chapter); and if you're wanting to lose weight check out the chapter "The Slimming Essentials."

Patchouli

(Pogostemon cablin)

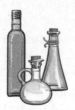

*Flowers . . . are a proud assertion that a
   ray of beauty
Outvalues all the utilities of the world.*
   —RALPH WALDO EMERSON

Patchouli is an essential oil that was popular in the 1970s, a free-wheeling era enjoyed by the love generation, perpetuated by hippies. Strong and sassy patchouli oil was a rite of passage, a fragrant flag that you wore to show you were part of the carefree, youth-oriented, anti-establishment movement. And hitchhiking while wearing the scent was like wearing a cowboy hat in a rural region. It was part of an era that has lingered on . . .

Standing on a highway and hitching a ride was an accepted pastime—and I did do this, both in my teens and mid-twenties. One weekend while on Highway 9 in the Santa Cruz mountains, a woman gave me a lift. A pungent, earthy aroma permeated the air in the van.

I asked, "What is that smell?"

The young natural-looking woman, who didn't wear makeup or fancy clothes, handed me a vial with a reddish-brown liquid in it. She removed the lid and dabbed the oil on my wrist.

"It's patchouli," she said.

At first, I developed a love/hate relationship with the pungent scent. Years later, I would wear it and like it for its fragrance. It acts as a symbol of connectedness to the planet, not just an oil that was used during the hippie movement in the sixties and seventies.

To this day, I wear patchouli, which is a casual and earthy scent that pairs well with blue jeans, a T-shirt, and boots. It's a distinct aroma that men more than women seem to be attracted to, perhaps because of its woodsy smell. When I do wear patchouli oil and go out, there is always a man (or two) that asks, "Is that patchouli?" It's like a code and a sign of approval that brings people together as it did in the twentieth century during change in America and around the world.

THE ROOTS OF PATCHOULI

Patchouli oil comes from India and it goes back five thousand years. It comes from the young leaves of an East Indian bush that boasts a strong scent due to exposure to air while the leaves are drying. After the distillation process, the oil goes from yellow to a dark reddish-brown—and it then has its telltale patchouli fragrance. This earthy oil also has roots in other Asian countries, including China and Taiwan. It enjoyed its resurgence in America and Europe during the sixties and seventies.

Aromatherapists will tell you this oil is pungent but earthy, and patchouli is an essential oil touted for its medicinal and aphrodisiac virtues. In the past, people of many cultures in both East and West countries used patchouli oil to perfume clothes and linen. I can attest in present-day, I have put a dab of the timeless patchouli oil on cloth jewelry braclets, and it leaves a musky, sensual fragrance.

Actually, there was a popular cologne I recall that my mother wore, and the small rectangular bottle that sat on the dresser in my parents' bedroom. Tabu cologne spray, a golden-colored liquid with a citrus and spicy fragrance was popular in the 1950s and '60s. It contains patchouli, cedarwood, clove, jasmine, orange, sandalwood, and other essential oils. But I was just a kid and didn't think about its ingredients. Ironically, I thought my mom was conventional, but it was a trendy fragrance during the hippie movement—and it is still available.

PATCHOULI ESSENTIALS

Patchouli oil is made of both leaves and stems; and like other essential oils, the extraction method is steam distillation. The compound called patchouli alcohol, which is a sesquiterpene alcohol, makes up perhaps more than half of the essential oil. This property makes it work as an anti-inflammatory, antidepressant, antiseptic, antioxidant, and sedative. Another percentage of the oil has antiviral properties, due to its alpha-bulnesene. And the oil's properties include alpha-guaiene, which has antidepressant, anti-inflammatory effects, and aphrodisiac benefits.

Yes, patchouli oil is believed to stimulate erotic feelings and it's likely due to its pheromone—the natural hormone that can enhance attraction.

Another compound in this essential oil is patchoulol, which is used in a cancer-treating chemotherapy drug called Taxol. It also contains germacene-B, a compound known for its antimicrobial and insecticide properties—both can be helpful, especially if you are in an area with annoying or deadly insects.

MEDICINAL POWERS OF PATCHOULI OIL

To help alleviate depression, the compound called patchouli alcohol can help boost mood like a natural antidepressant. When I wear a dab of patchouli oil on my wrist and run errands, I feel confident, sort of like wearing mascara or using a diffuser on my locks to give my hair volume. Yes, patchouli oil can help you feel oh-so good, naturally!

The aroma lessens appetite, which can essentially be a good thing for a myriad of reasons. If you're trying to lose unwanted pounds and body fat, patchouli can help you avoid overeating. Lovemaking, according to medical research, is known to have health virtues. Sex can help burn calories, boost your heart rate, reduce pain, and even help you to sleep better. So, due to the aphrodisiac potential qualities of patchouli oil, it can be healthful for both men and women.

This essential oil has many virtues, two being it is an antiseptic and antifungal, which can be used to treat skin ailments, from eczema to dry skin. It also has been used as a treatment for snakebites and insect stings.

Additional Advantages: The fragrance of distinct and unforgettable patchouli oil is believed to have a grounding influence on mood and confidence. It is often called an aphrodisiac because of its scent that is alluring to both men and women, which helps to boost self-confidence and self-esteem, important for overall mental well-being. I remember one late autumn afternoon, my neighbor, a younger man from San Francisco, said he knew I was in the backyard.

I hesitated but asked, "How?"

He answered, "The smell. I love the scent of the hippie oil."

And yes, a memorable affair followed with the guy next door.

Come On, Try It! It is used as a perfume, providing a calming effect for the body and spirit to feel grounded or centered. Patchouli can also be used in a compress diluted with a carrier oil to get its medicinal effects. It can be enjoyed in a diffuser, vaporizer, and incense form as well as beauty care, such as soaps. It is not a culinary essential oil.

Essential Safety Tip: Avoid internal use of patchouli essential oil.

The Feel-Good Moisturizer
Patchouli Earthy Cream

If you have ever had dry, dehydrated skin you know it loses its elasticity and can look and feel like a brown lizard's coat. Relieve rough skin with aromatherapeutic nutrients in this moisturizing lotion, which can be used and loved year-round, especially in the cold winters and hot summers, both of which can wreak havoc from head to toe. This recipe includes a combination of essential oils that complement patchouli, which has an intense fragrance.

14 drops rose essential oil
8 drops sandalwood essential oil
10 drops lavender essential oil
8 drops patchouli essential oil
½ ounce beeswax
4 ounces jojoba oil
3 ounces rose water

Combine oils together. Melt the beeswax and jojoba oil in a double boiler. Lower the heat and add the rose water slowly while beating the mixture. Remove from heat once you add the water. After cooling the mixture, add the essential oils. Use on hands, legs, feet, and any other dry parts of the body. You will look and feel like a reptile no longer!

Up next is another essential oil that you may be familiar with—at least as an ingredient in food and personal hygiene products. So get your adventurous attitude on because we're going back into the land of peppermint oil. Its popularity, past and present, as well as its versatility is why it's one oil that deserves plenty of kudos.

SCENT-SATIONAL HEALING OILS SHORT & SWEET

✓ Make a mental note that you can use patchouli oil as a quick go-to aphrodisiac due to its pheromone—the natural hormone that can enhance physical attraction to another person.
✓ To help zap mild depression, the compound called patchouli alcohol can help boost mood like a natural antidepressant . . .
✓ And jot down, when you're feeling balanced and calm due to the patchouli alcohol, it may enhance calmness and sleep.

✓ Patchouli also contains germacene-B, a compound known for its antimicrobial and insecticide properties—both can be helpful, especially if you live in or visit a region with insects that can bite or sting.

✓ Be aware researchers believe patchouli oil's properties of patchouli alcohol and alpha-guaiene, which both have anti-inflammatory properties, may help lower pain.

✓ Consider that this balancing down-to-earth essential oil may boost mood and help weight loss in other ways, too. (Refer to the chapter on slimming essentials to find out how this oil and other essential oils can help you to lose unwanted pounds.)

Peppermint

(Mentha piperita)

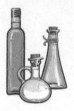

As for the garden of mint, the very smell of it alone recovers and refreshes our spirits, as the taste stirs up our appetite for meat.
—PLINY THE ELDER

When I was living in a tiny studio fit for a "pauper-ess," I worked as a coffee shop waitress on the graveyard shift—which came with peppermint oil to survive. One early morning, in the empty conference room while drinking peppermint tea, a co-worker took a vial out of her apron pocket.

"It's peppermint oil." She told me to take a sniff of it. "It works faster than sipping tea when you want energy."

Each shift my waitress friend shared the oil with me. It provided the extra boost I needed to get through the night-after-night.

I was balanced with better sleep, less pounds, and anticipating living in a real home and cooking and baking in a real kitchen. I gave thanks to the peppermint oil that helped give me stamina to carry on. To celebrate, I purchased my own bottle of peppermint oil, which I love to this day for getting me through the hard times.

THE ROOTS OF PEPPERMINT

I'm hardly alone savoring the gift of peppermint oil. History shows that the Romans crowned themselves with peppermint wreathes. Pliny, the scholar, said, "The very smell of it reanimates the spirit." This minty menthol oil is/was a popular essential oil because of its superior healing powers.

Asians, Egyptians, and Native Americans believed peppermint was a magical potion for an upset stomach. In the late eighteenth century, farmers in Europe began cultivating peppermint. No wonder the colonists brought peppermint to America.

As history goes, Smith Kerdon created Altoids in 1780 for stomach ailments. Pep O Mint Life Savers, a favorite mint candy in a roll, made their debut in the early twentieth century. As a kid in the 1960s, I recall my sister liked this variety, especially when going on a date with a boyfriend. In my early teens, I enjoyed my mom's semi-homemade peppermint coconut vanilla ice cream snowballs. These holiday treats were infused with crushed chocolate chips and a drop of peppermint oil. In the present-day, for a nostalgic feel during December, I recreate history with a twist by using store-bought gelato—a food on the Mediterranean food chart list—and put a drop of essential peppermint oil in dark chocolate gelato.

Peppermint Oil Has a Past

There are a variety of legends about the power of peppermint and its oil. As one legend goes, in Germany back in the late seventeenth century, a choirmaster for the Cologne Cathedral passed out peppermint sugar stick candy, which may have had the ingredient of mint oil like present-day peppermint sweets, to the young singers as an aid to keep them calm and quiet during the long ceremony. It was also said to celebrate the musical event the candies were shaped into shepherd's canes—like the red-and-white-striped kind we hung on our pine Christmas tree. Centuries later, nobody knows for sure the exact ingredients used in the peppermint candy canes (sugar would have given the children a quick burst of energy).

Interestingly, classic brands and types of peppermint candy from the twentieth century are still available today, including York Peppermint Patties and Altoids, which include oil of peppermint, an extract of the potent peppermint essential oil. So it could be possible oil of peppermint—or even a minute amount of the essential oil—was infused in the candy canes of yesteryear. After all, in the twenty-first century, some home bakers include peppermint essential oil for a mint flavor when baking cookies, cakes, and making candy.

Peppermint Essentials

Did you know that peppermint oil in your toothpaste comes from peppermint leaves and is extracted by steam distillation? What's more, peppermint is a hybrid of spearmint and watermint. The primary compound is menthol, which makes up more than half of the minty oil. And the other major component is menthone, a natural compound in peppermint oil as well as the floral geranium essential oil.

Menthol is a popular ingredient that is found in many medicinal products because of its variety of benefits. You may have noticed the strong scent and tingling feel in your mouth while sucking on a cough drop or cough syrup. Perhaps you've recognized the familiar aroma in a topical cream used for aches and pains. And like eucalyptus essential oil, menthol can be found in Vicks VapoRub to relieve congestion from a cold.

Other compounds in peppermint oil include 1,8 cinole (eucaluptol) like in basil essential oil, and methyl acetate, limonene, a-pinene, and b-pinene, which all contribute to its healing powers.

MEDICINAL POWERS OF PEPPERMINT OIL

Ever notice how mints are in a candy dish at the cash register when you walk out of a restaurant after a meal? Or perhaps you, like me, have sipped a cup of peppermint tea to help calm tummy troubles.

Peppermint oil may relieve stomach ailments by soothing the GI tract. Medical researchers report that essential peppermint oil, like the herbal tea, can help lessen nausea, too. It is believed menthol may be the key to why inhaling this oil can and does lessen nausea. One study published in the *Nursing* journal reports 123 people inhaled peppermint oil after cardiac surgery. They rated on a 1-to-5 scale in which "5" means nauseated. After inhaling the oil, two minutes later, the oil inhalers said their queasiness was lessened. The verdict: Essential peppermint oil for post-op nausea could be a first-line treatment. But more research is needed.[1]

Also, research shows that peppermint may help you to get better sleep. Have you seen the chocolate wrapped mint or two left on the pillow, especially in a luxury hotel? It is believed by people who tout folk remedies that peppermint oil acts as a muscle relaxant, which can help calm your nervous system.

Additional Advantages: Peppermint essential oil also can ease muscle pain due to its cooling effect, like eucalyptus essential oil. Health spa staff workers agree that essential peppermint oil provides healing powers. In particular it can act as an uplifting mood agent in treatments, such as facials, manicures, massages, and hydrotherapy. Also, the United States uses almost 10 million pounds of peppermint (and spearmint), and approximately 95 percent is used for candy, chewing gum, and toothpaste.[2]

Come On, Try It! Peppermint oil can act in different ways like a chameleon, the lizard that changes colors in a heartbeat. This mint oil can help you unwind and also be refreshing by using it in a diffuser or a quick spritz. You can consume one small drop neat (undiluted) under your tongue or dab one drop on your forehead or the back of your neck. It is another culinary essential oil and used in cooking and baking. Peppermint is used in body care treatments, including manicures, massage, and more.

Peppermint Honey Feet Treat

❖ ❖ ❖

Your feet are the foundation of your body, a podiatrist once told me. In graduate school when I was a server at many restaurants, after a long shift my feet were red and aching. To pamper my soles and swollen bunion, I would soak them in a bowl of hot water in hope of getting relief. Here is a natural remedy that includes peppermint essential oil to help lessen pain and inflammation, too.

4 tablespoons aloe vera gel
4 teaspoons grated beeswax
2 teaspoons honey
2 teaspoons fresh mint leaves (optional)
6 drops peppermint essential oil
2 drops arnica essential oil
2 drops camphor oil
2 drops eucalyptus essential oil

Rinse mint leaves and place on a paper towel to dry. Grind mint using coffee grinder (or by hand using mortar and pestle). Set aside. Melt beeswax using a small double boiler. In a microwave-safe glass bowl combine aloe vera and honey, mix well. Stir in beeswax. Let cool. Add mint and oils stirring until completely mixed. Apply after bath or shower to entire feet and toes. Store remaining Feet Treat in covered cool place away from sun or heat. Tip/Benefits: Aids in circulation of overworked feet. Moisturizes and softens while it soothes and restores tired aching feet. [Author's note: Personally, I recommend after 20 minutes, rinsing your feet with warm water as I did.]

(Courtesy: National Honey Board)

Out of the mint world, for now, and back into floral aromatherapy. One beautiful flower and its essential oil was not going to be ignored in this book. Yes, I'm talking about romantic rose oil, and its history and present-day uses may simply surprise you.

SCENT-SATIONAL HEALING OILS SHORT & SWEET

✓ Take note that peppermint essential oil is acknowledged around the world as a versatile healing medicine for the body.
✓ Scientists know menthol is a primary ingredient in peppermint—which can relieve congestion from a cold.
✓ Medical researchers have pinpointed that menthol can help to quell queasiness, and inhaling this oil can and does work fast.
✓ Also, research shows that peppermint may help enhance better sleep, perhaps due to its ability to soothe tummy trouble or aches and pains, which make it difficult to get good shut-eye.
✓ Be mindful that peppermint oil is found in lotions, shampoos, soaps, and candles, all of which can uplift your spirit and well-being.
✓ Don't forget, peppermint essential oil is a culinary oil and is used in toothpaste, mouthwash, dental floss, but also in baking—often infused in cakes, cookies, and candies.

Rose

(Rose centifolia)

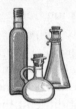

*True friendship is like a rose: we don't realize its
beauty until it fades.*
—EVELYN LOEB

I love rose oil . . . but my fondness comes from the rose petals—white, red, and pink. The floral fragrance is sublime, and rose oil is not excluded. One spring I was dating an older man. He was a globetrotter who introduced me to the world of roses, more than I had ever experienced. Each time he packed for an unaccompanied vacation, it was his mode of operation to lavish me with several bouquets of colorful roses. He would come to my rustic, Mediterranean-style bungalow in San Carlos, California, and act like a savvy and frugal real estate home stager.

Fascinated by his actions, I'd watch him take out vases in a discount store bag, and fill each one with water and a dozen on-sale, day-old roses. The fragrance was sweet and lingered in the air in each room. "By the time all these flowers turn brown," he said, "I'll be back home." While it was a romantic gesture, I felt sad watching the rose petals wilt.

My landlord, a surrogate grandmother and a wealthy woman, took pity on my plight of loneliness and the withering roses. One evening she paid me a visit. She gave me a vial filled with rose essential oil. She whispered, "This is expensive. But the beautiful thing is, the oil, unlike your man's cheap roses, will last longer." I treasured the rose oil. When I wore a dab of the oil on my wrist, I felt like a complete and natural woman without a man—a true gift to treasure.

THE ROOTS OF ROSE

Healing oil specialists will tell you rose oil has been noted way back in time—as far back as 5000 B.C. In Homer's *The Iliad*, Aphrodite anoints the body of Hector with rose oil. And rose water is an ancient Middle Eastern product, where rose petals were soaked in water, drained, and put into perfume, which came with a high price for its enjoyment.

It is interesting to note that since it takes three thousand to five thousand pounds of rose petals to make one pound of rose oil, it was not as widely used as other oils—the unusual high cost meant that people could not afford to buy it.[1]

As the legend is told by aromatherapists, Cleopatra put rose oil on a barge she traveled on, and the end result? She used this fragrant potion to attract Mark Antony. Evidently, the consensus is her resourceful usage of the floral oil lure did indeed woo and win the man she fancied.

ROSE ESSENTIALS

Romantic and pricey floral rose oil uses rose petals two ways: rose ottos are extracted by steam distillation, while rose absolutes are obtained through the solvent method. Rose oil contains many healing compounds, including a few that are superstars in other essential oils. Gerianol is believed to be nature's antidepressant. I cannot say if it is a cure-all for depression, but it may help boost your mood. Citral, an antimicrobial, can help fight germs, the culprits for flu, colds, infections, and superbugs.

Eugenol is also found in rose oil. It is a potent antioxidant, a disease fighter that can lower your odds of developing a weakened immune system, and even heart disease. Methyl eugenol, another compound in rose oil, is an antiseptic, which can be used to fight off germs. This strong arsenal of healing properties found in this floral essential oil can and does make rose essential oil a multipurpose tool.

Romantic Rose Oil Massage

A pampering massage can help relax you and your partner. Before a haircut gone wrong, I had promised to take my hungry mate out to a seafood restaurant on the water. Due to my embarrassment of the new look, I canceled. However, a day later I offered a dozen white roses as a peace offering. In hindsight, a mutual massage including rose oil would have been more appreciated, but I was young and naïve to the world of essential oil body work. This recipe is inspired by the lovely fragrant white rose.

1 ounce jojoba
1 ounce sweet almond oil
5 drops jasmine essential oil
10 drops rose essential oil
5 drops lemon essential oil
10 drops sandalwood essential oil
5 drops bergamot essential oil

Make a base oil with the jojoba and almond oils. Put in the essential oil and mix well. You can use this massage oil lightly from head to toe.

MEDICINAL POWERS OF ROSE OIL

Rose oil has a myriad of medicinal benefits. Its top healing powers include antidepressant benefits. So how exactly does rose oil help boost mood?

One pilot study published in the journal *Complementary Therapies in Clinical Practice* documented how twenty-eight postpartum women (think of the surrealistic film *Tully*, which shows the dark side after giving birth to a newborn), benefited from the use of rose oil. They were given a small blend of antidepressant geraniol rose oil and lavender oil twice a week for fifteen-minute intervals. The results: After one month there was a decline in depression, and anxiety, too.[2]

Also, other researchers believe rose oil may cause a decrease in breathing rate, blood oxygen saturation, and lower systolic blood pressure—all helping people to feel calmer. Two aromatic compounds, phenyl acetaldehyde and citronellyl acetate, could be responsible for stress relief due to the pleasant aroma of the floral essential oil. But more research is needed because pinpointing the exact compound in rose essential oil that may make it nature's antidepressant is still undecided—but geraniol is on the short list of potential properties that may be lessening depression.

Rose Otto, Practical Magic

Rose oil that is steam distilled is called "rose otto"; the extracted solvent is rose absolute. Rose essential oil is pricey; it can cost one hundred dollars for a small vial available online at essential oil companies. But there is an alternative way to gain access to it, says Lynda Ballard of Kobashi Essential Oils. Read on and let Lynda tell you how to get your rose and sniff it, too . . .

Rose Otto when blended in coconut oil is very affordable as the cost of pure rose otto is incredibly expensive, but well worth investing in for its truly heady and exquisite aroma. Known as "The Queen" of oils, it has an affinity

> with the female system and enjoyed a long history of use as a beauty aid. It is a great skin care oil helping with dry, mature skin and addressing the first signs of aging. We use rose otto in Kobashi facial massage oil, serum, lotion, and cream. A wonderful by-product of the distillation of rose is rose water. It contains the water-soluble elements of the plant, smells wonderful, and is a great skin tonic working well with the face oils and creams.

Additional Advantages: Rose oil also may be beneficial for libido. When men or women are anxious, inhibitions and feeling uneasy can get in the way of enjoying lovemaking. Rose oil's relaxing effect may be able to tackle these nerves. Rose oil is also used for skin care. Acne is often linked to hormonal fluctuations, during puberty, pre-menstrual syndrome, and menopause. When hormones go wild, rose oil may be helpful. Aromatherapists believe since rose oil provides antibacterial and antimicrobial benefits, it can be used to get rid of acne by using a drop undiluted on blemishes once or twice a day.

Come On, Try It! Rose essential oil is used in massage oils and lotions. The floral oil can be inhaled from the bottle or a drop or two put on a handkerchief to sniff. It also can be diluted with water and used in a vaporizer. Rose oil can be used in a blend for a bath. It is also available in soaps, shampoos, and even in foods.

Romance-Enhancing Lemon Pound Cake Squares with Rose Oil Glaze

In my childhood and young adult years I baked cakes, all kinds—cupcakes, sheetcakes, Bundt cakes, single and two-layer cakes. After the bad haircut saga, I adjusted to the new look, sort of, so I baked a cake as another forgiveness gesture for the mega meltdown my mate endured. If I could go back in time, I'd turn to nature's finest citrus oils, such as lemon topped with a "rose" for a fragrant imprint, making it romantic. This is my recipe that you should put to work when you need a peacemaker and there isn't enough time in the day. The cake is buttery and moist with an elegant, sweet rose oil glaze.

1 box premium pound cake mix
12 tablespoons butter, melted (save a teaspoon for
    greasing baking dish)
1 drop lemon oil

ROSE GLAZE

1 cup confectioners sugar
2–4 tablespoons organic half-and-half
1 drop rose essential oil
1 tablespoon honey
Fresh seasonal berries (blackberries or raspberries)

   Preheat oven to 350 degrees F. In a bowl, mix cake mix, butter, and lemon oil. Pour into an 8-inch by 8-inch butter-greased baking dish. Bake for approximately 45–55 minutes or until firm. Remove and cool. In a mixing bowl, combine sugar and half-and-half. Mix until creamy. Add rose oil and honey.*

Makes about 20 small squares.

*Use a toothpick to put a monitored drop of the oil. Drizzle with glaze. Top with berries. Serve with black or white tea, iced or hot depending on the season. Note: If you live in high altitude like I do, add 1 tablespoon all-purpose flour. Another option to glaze is homemade whipped cream with a drop of essential rose oil.

In the next pages, we're going to enter the land of herbal culinary essential oils once again. While rosemary is probably one of the most versatile and healing oils I dish up, it has plenty of surprising uses. Here comes an essential oil you don't want to be without in or out of the kitchen.

SCENT-SATIONAL HEALING OILS SHORT & SWEET

✓ Do comprehend that the compound geraniol may be nature's antidepressant and it's found in rose essential oil.

✓ And note, citral, an antimicrobial, can help fight germs which are the culprits for flu, colds, infections, and superbugs.

✓ Don't forget, eugenol also found in rose oil is a potent antioxidant, a disease fighter that can lower your odds of developing a weakened immune system, and even heart disease.

✓ Methyl eugenol, another compound in rose oil, is an antiseptic that can be used to fight germs.

✓ Rose oil used in a body massage, often a blend, can help you deplug and uplift your mood.

✓ You'll find costly rose essential oil is often blended with other oils and carrier oils to make it last longer when used in a variety of products, including beauty items, luxury spa treatments, and perfumes . . .

✓ And note, rose essential oil is an edible oil, used especially in sweet desserts like ice cream or frosting.

Rosemary

(*Rosmarinas officinalis*)

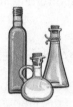

There's rosemary, that's for remembrance.
—WILLIAM SHAKESPEARE, *Hamlet*

Woodsy rosemary essential oil has a place in my heart and soul, tracing back to age fourteen when the Simon and Garfunkel tune "Scarborough Fair" played in my bedroom during the fall harvest moon. I recall savoring the aromas of parsley, sage, homemade rosemary oil, and thyme, as they rushed from my mom's simmering tomato sauce on the stovetop and permeated the air. As I grew up, whenever I heard the song it brought back memories of the rosemary-flavored entrées I savored at home.

Nowadays, I still use rosemary essential oil. It sits in my kitchen cabinet and enhances my Mediterranean entrées that I whip up using my mother's recipes. The scent often makes me nostalgic, as Shakespeare's words, "There's rosemary for remembrance" ring true.

THE ROOTS OF ROSEMARY

Rosemary, a refreshing, rejuvenating, and restorative essential oil was burned in shrines to symbolize loyalty. In the sixteenth century, the wealthy and the royalty who could afford such luxury essential oils filled their home with the aroma.

And rosemary was touted to have life-saving healing powers. It is one of the many herbs in the Thieves Formula, which was used to help prevent contracting the bubonic plague during the Middle Ages. These days, the biggest producers of rosemary oil are France and Spain, making it one more Mediterranean essential oil.

ROSEMARY ESSENTIALS

This ancient therapeutic herb has a woody and strong scent. Rosemary oil is extracted by steam distillation and solvent extraction, and comes from the flower tops and leaves. There are different varieties, one containing cineole and verbenone chemotypes, which is gentle in contrast to the camphor type.

Rosemary leaf holds the antioxidant pigment diosmin. Its other antioxidants include carnosol, carnosic acid, ursolic acid, rosmarinic acid, and caffeic acid. Research has been conducted looking at the chemical composition of these antioxidants found in rosemary essential oil from southern Spain. Rosemary also includes flavonoids, another disease-fighting antioxidant, and it has anti-inflammatory 1,8 cinole like calming chamomile essential oil.

MEDICINAL POWERS OF ROSEMARY OIL

Rosemary is believed to have many therapeutic benefits. Studies show that rosemary can help enhance memory to boost the nervous system that helps boost energy. Aromatherapists believe massaging the oil or using the essential oil topically combined with a carrier oil on the skin may also lessen inflammation due to its antioxidants as well as to help ease aching muscles.

Past research at Penn State shows that rosemary can do more with its antioxidants. In fact, it may reduce the risk of developing cancer.

But the jury is still out until a human-controlled study or more findings in lab research (think petri dishes and earthshaking conclusions) are conducted.

The aromatherapy effects are good for respiratory ailments, including lung congestion. While this essential oil has good health benefits, it is also used as a sensual oil thanks to its refreshing fragrance that can boost your spirits.

Additional Advantages: Rosemary oil is touted for its ability to enhance alertness and heightened brainpower. It can help your mind to focus, alleviate brain fog, and make it easier to concentrate on mental tasks.

Come On, Try It! Rosemary essential oil has an herbal aroma that can be used for massages and baths. It is also used in hair products, cosmetics, and bath products such as soaps and gels. You can also enjoy this oil in food since it is an essential culinary oil used for both savory and sweet dishes paired with entrées to desserts.

Healing
California Dreaming
Rosemary, Thyme, Parsley Spaghetti

❖ ❖ ❖

I revisited Monterey, California, imagining it would be the same as it was decades ago. Well, things change. Trying to find a hotel in Pacific Grove was a task while driving in circles amid traffic. Once there, it was my fantasy to go to Cannery Row, the place noted by my favorite author John Steinbeck. Also, I wanted to enjoy a hot meal, such as Cioppino with herbal flavors like rosemary and garlic. However, to avoid the crowded restaurants on a Saturday night, I ended up munching on cold French fries in the rustic hotel room. I vowed to cook an aromatic feast using culinary essential oils back home.

The highlight of the trip was on the way home stopping at a roadside produce stand in Moss Landing. It was there I stocked up on gigantic tomatoes and garlic—perfect to make the aromatic meal of my dream. Back home I cooked up this California coast–inspired rosemary oil–infused pasta sauce and spaghetti to make up for the herbal dinner with an ocean view I didn't get to have.

½ cup extra virgin oil
¼ cup garlic cloves and yellow onion, minced
6 Roma tomatoes, chopped
1 tablespoon fresh thyme
Ground black pepper and sea salt to taste
1 drop rosemary essential oil
2 cups whole grain spaghetti, cooked
Parmesan cheese, shavings
Parsley (garnish)
Old country Italian bread, fresh
European-style butter or olive oil (for dipping bread)
Fresh parsley, chopped (for garnish)

In a deep skillet on medium heat place extra virgin olive oil, garlic, and onions. Lightly sauté for a few minutes. Add tomatoes, thyme, pepper, and salt. Turn to simmer. Cook about 25 minutes until the tomatoes turn into a chunky sauce texture. Add just 1 drop of rosemary essential oil. While the sauce is simmering, cook pasta per box directions. When al dente, remove. Place pasta on plates, top with sauce. Sprinkle with cheese and parsley. Serve with slices of warm bread and real butter or dip in olive oil.

Serves 2 or 3.

Now that I've put rosemary on the kitchen table, it's time to bring out another essential oil—one that blends well with other culinary herb oils. Let's take a look at sage and find out things that may surprise you.

SCENT-SATIONAL HEALING OILS SHORT & SWEET

✓ The antioxidant compounds in rosemary essential oil may help lower the risk of developing heart disease.

✓ By adding antioxidant-rich rosemary to tomato sauce rich in the antioxidant lycopene—it can help strengthen the immune system.

✓ Rosemary essential oil adds flavor to savory dishes, like pasta plates and shellfish soups, part of a Mediterranean heart-healthy diet.

✓ And rosemary essential oil can be used in cooking and baking, which makes it budget-friendly and convenient to use year-round since the herb is not always available fresh and is more flavorful than dried.

Sage

(Salvia officinalis)

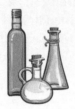

The garden should be adorned with roses and lilies,
the turnsole violets, and mandrake; there you
should have parsley, cost fennel, southern wood,
coriander, sage, savory hyssop, mint, rue,
dittany, small age, pellitony, lettuces, garden trees,
and peonies.
—ALEXANDER OF NECKHAM,
Of the Nature of Things, 1187

Back to the Bay Area Peninsula, I spent time working as a transient journalist in the San Francisco Bay Area. On an assignment, it was my job to interview two middle-aged notorious men who owned a night-club in San Francisco. The dynamic duo had a surprise waiting for me at a restaurant in North Beach. We walked into a cozy Italian restaurant complete with white and red tablescapes, waiters, and French bread placed on the tables. I was overcome with the seductive smell of Mediterranean cuisine.

Once at our table, sitting with menus, a hefty man with a patch over his eye sat down with us. I was introduced to him—a well-known "S.F. Chronicle" columnist. I didn't know who he was; and my face turned red when I was told by my subject, just as our sage pasta dish was served. Now, when I use sage oil in my pasta dishes—I recall the familiar smell and the columnist's name.

THE ROOTS OF SAGE

The roots of sage, also called garden sage, common sage, and culinary sage, go back centuries. It may have originated in the Mediterranean countries. Known as a superior camphor-flavored "fountain of youth" herb, its leaves are extracted to make essential sage oil. Its Latin name means "to heal or save."

In ancient times, Greeks and Romans believed sage to be a sacred herb. And, as the legend goes, sage, all forms, will enhance longevity if used on a regular basis. Ancient Egyptian women turned to sage in hope of bearing children, whereas the Greek doctor Dioscorides found sage could be used to treat coughs.

There are different versions of the Four Thieves Formula, but some of them did include healing sage oil as one of the ingredients. As time passed, sage oil was used to preserve food since refrigeration had not been discovered. It was also used to flavor foods, including Italian cuisine and French, who used it in their variety of meats.

SAGE ESSENTIALS

Sage, like most of the essential oils in my picks, comes from leaves and flowers and is extracted by steam distillation. There is sage and clary sage, which is another variety of the popular essential oil but it isn't believed to have the exceptional antiseptic qualities. The essential oils, sage and clary sage, are sold separately by their names. Sage oil has a sharp, herbal aroma, which contains healing properties.

The primary compounds include the main antibacterial compounds, including a-pinene, camphene, camphor, b-pinene, nyrcene, and limonene—which may help to lessen the risk of developing inflammation, fight fungal infections, and even protect against microbes.

MEDICINAL POWERS OF SAGE OIL

In the twenty-first century, viruses and bacterial infections are contracted wherever you go, be it at the workplace, store, airplane, or even your home. Sage essential oil and its protective compounds may help guard you from catching a virus or flu—deadly even in the present day.

Epidemics can and do happen in real life. Making a spray or lotion including sage oil isn't a bad idea. Note to self: Bring a sage spray before entering hotel rooms when traveling, and at home after being around people.

Additional Advantages: Aromatherapists and herbalists claim sage is nature's antiseptic and astringent. Its healing powers are much more than that, though. This essential oil can be used in a variety of ways. It can be both calming and stimulating. It's a good oil to use in massages to relax muscles.

Come On, Try It! Sage oil has an herbal smell and has both antiseptic and antifungal uses. It can be put in a vaporizer to zap germs and fight viruses. You can use it diluted with a carrier oil such as olive oil directly on blemishes or cuts and scrapes. Sage is also a culinary essential oil.

Fragrant and Savory
Sage Cheese Cornbread

❖ ❖ ❖

Cornbread is a common quick bread in America. Years ago, I used to buy a convenient store-bought mix of honey cornbread that boasts on the package "natural." One day an acquaintance of mine was shocked that I didn't make this bread from scratch. "You used a box mix?" Her harsh words made me pause. Her comment was like that sound you hear when accidentally scraping your fingernail on a blackboard. So, yeah, it was an aha moment that made me go back to making homemade cornbread with an essential oil twist.

This batch of cornbread is my recipe inspired by California herbs. Making this bread from scratch is almost as easy as the box stuff, but it smells even better in your kitchen and your palate will thank you.

1 cup all-purpose flour
1 cup cornmeal
1 tablespoon baking powder
¼ cup sugar
1 large organic egg
¾ cup buttermilk
¼ cup orange juice (squeeze from an orange)
⅓ cup European-style butter or extra virgin olive oil
*   (save a bit to grease the dish)*
1 drop lemon essential oil
1 drop sage essential oil
Raw honey and butter (for honey butter)

In a medium bowl, mix dry ingredients (flour, cornmeal, baking powder, and sugar). Add wet ingredients (egg, buttermilk, juice, and butter or oil). Add essential oil. Pour batter into lightly buttered 8-inch by 8-inch dish. Bake at 400 degrees F for about 25 minutes or until firm and light golden brown. Cool. Serve warm. (Mix equal parts of honey and butter for a cream honey butter.) You can slice squares from the dish or turn it over and out on a cutting board. Serve on a dish or bread basket.

Serves 10 to 12.

I've put sage in my essential oils lockbox, and hopefully it's in yours, too, expanding your collection. And now it's time to bring in another oil—one that is an all-time darling of mine. Let's take a look at sandalwood, used in earthy body oils, incense, and much more.

SCENT-SATIONAL HEALING OILS SHORT & SWEET

✓ Sage may help bolster the immune system because of its antibacterial compounds, including a-pinene and limone.

✓ Rosemary and sage culinary oils are both antioxidant-rich and can complement Mediterranean foods, including soups, stews, and breads for heart health and flavor.

✓ Sage oil can be budget-friendly in contrast to using fresh sage.

✓ Safely consumed in tiny portions, adding to recipes can be an ideal addition to a Mediterranean Diet and lifestyle.

Sandalwood

(Santalum album)

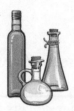

*If I had a place made of pearls, in land with jewels,
scented with musk, saffron and sandalwood, a sheer
delight to behold—seeing this, I might go astray
and forget You, and Your name would not enter my
mind.*

—SRI GURU GRANTH SAHIB

One spring I was cautious to take the ferry ride from Long Beach to
Catalina Island, despite using the ancient Buddhism regimen of
putting sandalwood oil on my wrist for staying calm and alert. I wasn't
convinced the sandalwood potion would rescue me, so once boarding
the ferry I fled to the bathroom. My refuge was sitting on the com-
mode in the stall as I waited for the huge swells to capsize the boat. I
waited. I waited. "When will the monster swells hit?" I wondered. But
nothing happened. The voyage was smooth sailing, no big breakers.

Perhaps, the sandalwood oil remedy kept me grounded, too. The Zane Grey Pueblo Hotel overlooking Avalon Bay was the prize and I reaped the rewards of staying at the Hopi Indian styled abode. I stayed in the famous late Western author's study complete with an outdoor swimming pool, hotel cats, and the calming scent of sandalwood incense.

On the ferry again, a sniff of sandalwood oil was my tried-and-true antidote. Like Rose's character in the *Titanic* film scene, I stood on the bow of the boat (well, maybe I tilted my head downward over the rim of the vessel) overlooking the water. The essential oil scent was relaxing, a bit like Dr. Clower must feel when sailing his boat on calm water and smelling the sea air.

THE ROOTS OF SANDALWOOD

This woody, musky, earthy oil has been used by Buddhists in religious rituals and other religious events for over four thousand years. Sandalwood incense was also used in Indian temples to help worshippers relax while meditating. The Polynesians used sandalwood to cure headaches and heal skin ailments, which isn't surprising because of this essential oil's multitude of healing compounds.

The history of sweet sandalwood oil includes its being known as an aphrodisiac and was often used in the Eastern world. The Arabian doctor Avicenna believed it could "heal passions of the heart."[1]

Sandalwood oil is known to be used in religious rituals, including Buddhism, Hinduism, Sufism, as well as Chinese, Japanese, and Korean ceremonies. I have a twenty-year-old small white ceramic item, which is a single Buddha man. It is used for burning incense. And yes, sandalwood incense cones have been burned in it for years. It sits in a Zen-like group—a white ceramic cat, and white tea pot set on an antique glass table in the dining room.

SANDALWOOD ESSENTIALS

Sandalwood is most commonly extracted by steam distillation. It comes from the heartwood and roots. But other methods of extraction, including water and solvent, have been used, too. It contains santalol, which makes up the majority of the oil. This component is believed to help achieve optimum oxygen levels in the bloodstream, and like calming lavender essential oil is beneficial for relieving anxiety. It can also boost a restful state leading to a good night's sleep thanks to its melatonin.

Case-in-point, when I moved to the Sierra Nevada, living in a cold climate complete with snowstorms and power outages was stressful to me—at first. I recall purchasing packets of sandalwood incense sticks during those chilly winter nights. The wood scent relaxed me at bedtime. I used to wear sandalwood body oil at night when enjoying North Beach nightlife in San Francisco. In the mountains, though, I paired sandalwood essential oil with jojoba oil and dabbed it on my wrist.

Other healing compounds in sandalwood essential oil are santyl acetate and santalenes. "It's antibacterial, antiviral, antifungal," explains aromatherapist Sascha Beck adding, "*and* it calms the nervous system."

MEDICINAL POWERS OF SANDALWOOD OIL

First and foremost, sandalwood oil is touted for its anti-inflammatory health benefits. Past research has shown that sandalwood essential oil provides relief from all types of inflammation, including digestive disorders, nerves, and circulatory issues.

Researchers have observed that santalol has been shown to halt cytokine and chemokine cells, two key markers of inflammation. It's believed that sandalwood essential oil, because of this compound, acts like the over-the-counter anti-inflammatory medicine ibuprofen.

Other health benefits of sandalwood oil include staving off coughs and sore throats, boosting your memory, and acting as an antiseptic for cuts and wounds. Not only is sandalwood used in medicines, but also it can be an ingredient in healing skin care.

Additional Advantages: Karlis C. Ullis, M.D., a retired sports doctor in Pacific Palisades, California, touts the merits of sandalwood oil, too. "I use sandalwood as a deodorant. Plus, it produces an erotic feeling," he told me. Dr. Ullis added, "I use the one from India—a pure oil. It is used widely in Hindu wedding ceremonies." He buys the personal hygiene item from both India and at Indian shops in town. Dr. Ullis shared that the oil is known to be erotic for married couples and can battle the heat due to its cooling effect.

Beck added: "The oil's anti-inflammatory properties assist with inflamed and dry skin conditions. My favorite use is to blend it with other essential oils in a face potion."

Come On, Try It! This earthy oil also can be enjoyed with a carrier oil like almond oil and used as a confidence-boosting body perfume or in a destressing massage or bath. It can also be inhaled from a diffuser, vial, incense, or candle to help you to relax and feel more at ease with yourself and others.

Calming and Comforting Sandalwood Massage Oil

One night in the San Francisco Bay Area, during a dating phase, my companion arrived at my bungalow with a bag. Curious, I asked him what was inside.

"A surprise," he answered.

After a film and dinner, I was greeted by the mystery item inside the bag. It was a sandalwood blend massage oil, which smelled like the fresh cut pine wood I used to make a salad bowl in my high school woodshop class. I was treated to a romantic massage. In retrospect, I will say the aroma was the most sensual part of that night because it took me back in time. I was the only girl in class and attracted a lot of male attention and help working on wood projects. I received an A grade. However, when it was my turn to reciprocate a massage—I failed. Honestly, I was clueless on what to do but I made a note to self: Read a book on the art of massage. This recipe is dedicated to lovers or to those wanting to fall in love or feel alive smelling nature's odor.

10 drops rose essential oil
10 drops sandalwood essential oil
5 drops jasmine essential oil
5 drops lavender essential oil
1 ounce jojoba oil

Mix your essential oils together. Add to the jojoba carrier oil. Blend well. Apply a small amount into your hand, swirl the oil around, and massage onto your partners' body parts, including arms, back, and legs.

As you near the end of my chosen essential oils, another minty oil is up next. Discover all the reasons, like I did, why it is a valuable essential oil. You won't be surprised it made the short list!

SCENT-SATIONAL HEALING OILS SHORT & SWEET

✓ Sandalwood oil may help reduce inflammation because it contains santalol, which can block two key inflammation markers.
✓ This woody essential oil has more sesquiterpenes than most essential oils . . .
✓ This, in turn, means inhaling sandalwood may help boost oxygen levels in the bloodstream, and can create a calming effect.
✓ And it can relax you during a massage, so sandalwood is often used in spa body treatments. Plus, its properties can enhance your spirit.

Spearmint

(Mentha spicata)

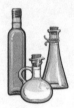

A man in all the world's new fashion planted,
That hath a mint of phases in his brain.
—WILLIAM SHAKESPEARE, *Love's Labour's Lost,*
Act 1, Scene 1

One holiday season, I was seeing the easy on the eyes man from San Francisco who gave me the sandalwood sensual massage. We had a connection due to our mutual love of writing. And then we began to spend time together, working out at the local gym, and sipping tea at night. Then, the day after Christmas I received the news.

"I got my dream job!" I was elated until I heard the next sentence. "It's in New York."

My heart sank. The soul mate of *my dreams* was moving three thousand miles away. He gifted me with a eucalyptus and spearmint body wash. My sibling poked fun at the present and called it, "a stupid bar of soap." But this healing token was so much more to me . . .

In my mind, I created a symbolic deadline. "I will use this soap," I vowed. "Once it is gone, if I don't hear from him—I'll move on." A week passed. No word. Weeks passed and the minty, tingling wash was almost gone like a fading love.

Late that evening, the phone rang. I heard the familiar voice and three words, "I miss you."

It was him! I could smell the mint on my hands that once held his. While we never saw each other again, memories of our affair left me with a fondness for the aroma of spearmint oil and it makes me smile to this day.

THE ROOTS OF SPEARMINT

Spearmint is derived from the Mediterranean countries. Ancient Egyptians, Greeks, and Romans were believed to have used it for centuries. Spearmint, the plant, was noted by Pliny, the Roman herbalist. Spearmint was used in dozens of concoctions for its benefits for digestion.

Both peppermint and spearmint are the two most popular mints in the past and present day. As a kid growing up in the fifties and sixties, spearmint oil was very much around. My mom used the oil to make lamb chops paired with a mint sauce. I chewed Wrigley's spearmint gum and watched my big sister make love chains with the wrappers.

Brach's Spearmint candy was also familiar to me. Spearmint toothpaste, flavored with the oil, greeted me every morning and night. And spearmint jelly leaf-shaped candies filled a pretty scalloped candy dish that sat on a dining room table in our next-door neighbor's home.

SPEARMINT ESSENTIALS

The essential oil is extracted from the spearmint's leaves through steam distillation like the majority of my top 20 essential oil picks. Like peppermint oil, spearmint is minty but it has a gentler scent and flavor. It's sweeter as well. Spearmint essential has a pale yellow to greenish hue. But don't let its softer side fool you into thinking it isn't a powerful essential oil. It packs a punch of constituents.

Its mighty components include a-pinine, b-pinine, carvone, lina-

lool, limonene, 1,8 cinole, and a small amount of menthol and myrcene. It's the mix of these ingredients that gives spearmint its power
to work as an antiseptic and antispasmodic and so much more!

MEDICINAL POWERS OF SPEARMINT OIL

These days, essential oils from aromatic plants are used for stomach bugs. Medical research shows that spearmint essential oil may
fight bacteria. A Pakistan study published in the *Journal of Essential
Oil Research* shows spearmint oil's antimicrobial function may be due
to its compounds cis-carveol and carvone. Other studies show it can
attack *Escherichia coli.*[1]

Also, spearmint and peppermint oils may be beneficial for cancer
symptoms linked to chemotherapy side effects, such as nausea,
which could also be helpful for anything from travel sickness to pre-
menstrual symptoms. Medical researchers discovered both spearmint
and peppermint oils are recommended for their antispasmodic effects
on the stomach. In a study using capsules filled with two drops of
each oil, people dealing with chemotherapy nausea experienced improved results and had less queasiness.[2]

Spearmint essential oil is frequently used in toothpaste, which I
personally believe gives it a cleansing feel and a nice taste that lingers
in the mouth. It's not rocket science that good dental hygiene is essential to our good health, well-being, and appearance, too. If you
have gum disease the odds are increased that heart disease may become a problem.

Additional Advantages: Spearmint oil doesn't stop there. It's also useful for better digestion, boosting the spirit, treating headaches, muscle aches and pains, and stress. You can use spearmint essential oil by
sniffing it or ingesting it. Due to the components noted, it can help
calm an upset stomach since it also reduces cramps.

Come On, Try It! Spearmint oil can be used topically with a carrier oil
for skin conditions such as acne. It is used in personal hygiene products, from toothpaste and dental floss, to shampoo and soap. It's also
added into massage oil blends. You can use it in cooking and even in a
cup of tea or a glass of water.

Refreshing and Calming
Double Mint-Flavored Water

I usually drink store-bought spring water. It all started one summer day, when I opened up a letter stating our mountain water contained arsenic. I went to the grocery store and I purchased bottled water...and haven't stopped since that day. However, sometimes I crave flavored water. One afternoon I didn't have fresh mint but I did have a new bottle of spearmint essential oil. This simple beverage is inspired by my love for flavorful water, keeping me and you hydrated and heathier.

16 ounces water, bottled or filtered
Fresh lemon slices
1 teaspoon honey
1 drop spearmint essential oil
Ice cubes
Mint leaves for garnish

In a tall glass pour water, add citrus, honey, spearmint oil and stir. Add ice. Top with mint.

Tip: when using essential oils in tea, coffee, or water, mix well to keep the oil from rising to the top. Honey does not dilute the oil, but it can sweeten your beverage.

Serves 2.

Now that you've got the basics of spearmint oil and its versatile uses—it's time to bring on board another popular essential oil that is a must-have year-round. Tea tree oil gets kudos for its multiple healing powers, and you're going to find out just how versatile it is!

SCENT-SATIONAL HEALING OILS SHORT & SWEET

✓ Check out the variety of spearmint essential oil components, including a-pinine, limonene, and menthol, which give it the power to work as an antiseptic and antispasmodic.

✓ Spa treatments such as body massages and facials include spearmint oil due to its menthol effect that can be invigorating and increase blood circulation . . .

✓ And getting the blood flowing can help make you feel more energetic and lower the risk of heart disease.

✓ Spearmint essential oil is also used in dental products, which act as an antiseptic to fight bacteria—a cause of dental caries and gum disease.

✓ Don't ignore drinking water—and adding a bit of spearmint oil will help flavor up bland H_2O in the wintertime (when our thirst is less than summer months) to stave off the risk of dehydration—a key issue for everyone, especially the elderly.

Tea Tree

(Melaleuca alternifolia)

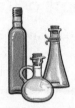

*Plants are the young of the world, vessels of health
and vigor; but they grope ever towards upward
consciousness.*
> —RALPH WALDO EMERSON, "Nature"

I do favor woodsy and citrus essential oils, but medicinal oils, from eucalyptus to tea tree, are a must for irksome health ailments. During a muscle-building phase, my regimen five days per week included walking five miles round-trip to a gym and cross-training with free weights and aerobics. After the hour of fitness, I'd treat myself to a sauna and a shower. Then, I'd make the trek back home while wearing sneakers without socks. One day I noticed my feet were red, flaky, and itchy. Athlete's foot. I recalled the fitness instructor who saw me scowl at my scaly lizard-like toes; she recommended tea tree oil to get rid of the unattractive and annoying ailment.

Tempted to go to the drugstore and buy an over-the-counter cream, I went to the health food store. I brought home a bottle of the tea tree oil and got a foot spa bath massager with heat, and bubbling water jets. Each night I soaked my achy, itchy red feet in a foot bath, and used a blend of tea tree and lavender essential oils. Not only did the bubbling water soothe my feet but the fragrance was calming. One week later: My red, itchy feet were history. I treated myself to a manicure and a pampering pedicure.

THE ROOTS OF TEA TREE

In 1770, when Captain Cook landed at Botany Bay, his men used tea tree leaves, which is what the oil is derived from, in a drink. It is believed the tea tree helped restore their health, curing skin infections and inflammation. Tea tree oil was commercialized back in the 1920s when Arthur Penfold, an Australian, saw business potential in the native essential oil. He believed tea tree oil showed promise due to its antiseptic properties.[1]

Also, in the twentieth century, tea tree oil was popular for its antibacterial, antiviral, and antifungal healing powers. During World War II, soldiers used tea tree oil to heal wounds. In the mid-century, however, antibiotics became the drug of choice and tea tree oil was put on the back burner. In the seventies, the potent tea tree oil made a comeback, especially with people living in impoverished countries, because it is less expensive than antibiotics.

In the twenty-first century, tea tree essential oil grew popular again, among aromatherapists to medical researchers who have studied the oil for decades. Its compounds make it an effective oil to use for a variety of health ailments that can be tended to at home.

TEA TREE ESSENTIALS

As with other essential oils, tea tree has two different varieties; one is niaouli, which has antiviral compounds and a more pleasing aroma, and cajeput, which smells harsher. Again, the oil comes from the flower tops and is extracted by steam distillation.

Medical research shows tea tree oil contains antimicrobial and anti-inflammatory properties called terpinen-4-ol and a-terpinol. These two components may help fight diseases linked to bacteria, infection, and inflammation—a big culprit in the world of health ailments. Also, the medicinal oil contains 1,8-cinole, a-terpinene, a-pinene, limonene, and linalool.

The compounds in tea tree essential oil are plentiful. With its medicinal odor, like eucalyptus, you'll learn to love it for its benefits, which outweigh the sterile and strong medicinal aroma. Nope, it's not sweet-smelling like rose or a forest-like aroma of Sandalwood essential oils—its fragrance is pungent, like a sterile scent in a dental office but one that you know after using it that it is going to help heal what's ailing you.

MEDICINAL POWERS OF TEA TREE OIL

This essential oil is an extremely versatile medicinal wonder with plenty of scientific studies to back up its benefits. It's touted to fight bacteria and viruses, including the common cold and the flu. Also, it's nature's immunity booster since it boosts white blood cells, which are important to keep you healthy.

Tea tree oil is an all-purpose oil used for multiple home cures, including acne, athlete's foot, nail fungus, rashes, insect bites, and wounds. It's a universal infection-fighting oil that can help reduce inflammation. It is an essential oil to have in your medicine cabinet and one of the top oils to have for all seasons.

Additional Advantages: This potent oil can be effective as a mouthwash, and to treat canker and cold sores. Its properties terpinen-4-ol and a-terpinol can help lessen severity of inflammation and potential infection. Tea tree oil has a strong smell and is a good cure-all for fighting germs.

Come On, Try It! It can be used directly on the skin but diluted is advised. It can also be used in an essential oil blend diluted with water and/or a carrier oil for foot baths, and even in a vaporizer or diffuser. Tea tree oil can be enjoyed in a massage oil blend with a carrier oil, too. But note, it is not a culinary oil.

Essential Safety Tip: Tea tree oil has been used as a mouth rinse, but caution is recommended. Unlike a saltwater oral rinse, it should never be swallowed.

Natural Freshener
Tea Tree–Lemon Air Disinfectant

My sibling started driving Uber for part-time income, which can be lucrative in a busy tourist town. The downfall? He showed me the can of anti-germ spray he used after each ride was completed. I read the long list of ingredients, alerting me the can was chock-full of toxic chemicals. I darted, covering my nose.

There had to be a more natural way to clean the air. At home, I turned to a DIY air spray for the cabin thinking I could get sick from his riders, too. This tea tree and lemon combo contains antibacterial compounds and is a natural disinfectant. Not only does it clean stale air, but it's invigorating to the mind and spirit, too.

1 drop tea tree essential oil
1 drop lemon essential oil
½ cup water

Put essential oils and water into an essential oil diffuser. I purchased one online. After cleaning the bathroom, where the cat box is, or kitchen after cooking and cleaning up, this tea tree–lemon spray smells wonderful, light, and cleansing. After I turn off the diffuser, I empty the container, per instructions. You can also put the ingredients in a spray bottle and spritz the air around you. (Use 8 ounces of water.)

So now you've got one more essential oil to add to your stock. The last essential oil coming up is one of my much loved scents. It is a sweet and comforting oil often used in a blend for beauty or culinary delights. I love this last top oil—and you may, too, once you learn more about it.

SCENT-SATIONAL HEALING OILS SHORT & SWEET

✓ Know that tea tree oil contains antimicrobial and anti-inflammatory properties called terpinen-4-ol and a-terpinol. These two components may help fight diseases linked to bacteria, infection, and inflammation . . .

✓ And inflammation is a primary cause of health ailments. But this essential oil can help lessen redness and swelling when used topically.

✓ And note, tea tree oil used on unsightly blemishes, itchy athlete's foot, and painful insect bites can be helpful to lessen pain and speed up the healing process.

✓ The lesson: Do not go barefooting in a locker room, *and* if you do suffer from athlete's feet—which is contagious—turn to therapeutic tea tree oil for a quick healing home cure.

✓ While tea tree oil can be used topically it should never be swallowed . . .

✓ And, of course, remember that tea tree oil should not be used as a culinary oil.

Vanilla

(Vanilla plantifolia)

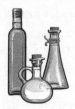

The centuries last passed have also given the taste important extension; the discovery of sugar, and its different preparations, of alcoholic liquors of wine, ices, vanilla, tea and coffee, have given us flavors hitherto unknown.

—JEAN ANTHELMO BRILLAT-SAVARIN

One morning, I waited for a woman to interview me, a city girl who likes getting regular manicures and getting highlights done at a hair salon, as a prospective tenant in her Lake Tahoe rental ranch home. I wanted to make her visit homey, so I put a bowl of vanilla essential oil–scented potpourri on the coffee table. The view from my upstairs home was breathtaking—one could view the cool fog above the San Carlos hills—a painted vision, much like a Monet painting. But despite this, and the warm, sweet aroma of vanilla floating in the air, the meeting was awkward.

I sat on the floor next to the old-time floor heater. The elderly lady scrutinized me like I was a slug on a slab in biology class. Inhaling the vanilla potpourri, admiring my fresh French painted pedicure stand out on the cold wood floor, I heard her forecast.

"You won't make it more than a month," she predicted.

The end result: I moved into a seventy-year-old cabin, complete with wood paneling, high beam ceilings, fireplace, and surrounded by pine trees. Twenty years later . . . I've weathered the Snow Armageddon of 2017, earthquake swarms, wildfires, bears, and wild raccoons camping in the fireplace—all by inhaling comforting vanilla essential oil. The familiar sweet fragrance calms and connects me to my Mediterranean-style home that lives on in my heart, despite losing it to gentrification.

The Roots of Vanilla

The history of vanilla essential oil goes back centuries. It was cultivated in countries like Tahiti and Java. The Spaniard Cortez is given credit for introducing the spice to Europe. When explorers docked on the Gulf Coast of Mexico, vanilla was called *vaina*, which meant "little pod."

In the past it was used in aromatherapy, including the use of massage, candles, incense, and even perfume, bubble bath, and soap. Not only has vanilla essential oil been used for beauty and aromatherapy, but it has a history for its calming benefits as well as being an aphrodisiac.

Vanilla Essentials

The bean pod is used to create the essential oil, which is extracted by the solvent CO_2 method like other absolute oils. Not unlike the other essential oils I have shared with you, vanilla contains good-for-you antioxidants that can enhance the immune system.

The main component of vanilla is vanillin, which is the most essential component of the two hundred or more compounds in vanilla beans. This light-colored, sweet-smelling oil also boasts antibacterial properties, due to its eugenol and vanillin zaldehyde—these two compounds may help fight infection. And that's not all... [1]

Vanilla Absolute Oil

People get confused when understanding what vanilla essential oils is and that it is not edible like vanilla extract or vanilla paste. Vanilla oil is very potent so it must be used with a carrier oil. Also, vanilla absolute should not be consumed. However, vanilla extract, which contains a lot of the healing compounds that vanilla absolute does, is ideal for sweet dishes like cakes, cookies, ice cream, and scones. And, yes, vanilla absolute does provide an aroma and properties to aid health and well-being.

MEDICINAL POWERS OF VANILLA OIL

Due to its antioxidant power, vanilla essential oil has been noted in the scientific world as a potential aid to help lower the risk of developing cancer. A study published in the *Journal of Agricultural and Food Chemistry* notes both vanilla extract and the essential oil contain many of the same antioxidant compounds that possibly may help inhibit the growth of cancer cells in breast and lung cancer. [2]

Vanilla essential oil may also keep your blood pressure on an even keel. The calming effect of the oil's vanillin may lower blood pressure because it calms the mind and body and lessens stress, which can overlap with anxiety and depression, too. In one study published in the *Indian Journal of Pharmacology*, it was discovered that vanillin showed antidepressant action in rodents. More research is needed but for now, research and anecdotal evidence shows promise in boosting mood. [3]

Medical researchers and aromatherapists will tell you vanilla essential oil, thanks to its antioxidants, may help dilated arteries and fight damage to blood vessels. Vanilla essential oil can lower the risk of developing cancer and heart disease, but it has even more powers to offer to you.

Additional Advantages: Vanilla essential oil aids in inflammation linked to fever, and this is due to eugenol and vanillin. It has been known to help reduce insomnia, aches, and pains from arthritis. Also, calming vanilla can help stave off PMS anxiety to menopause stress, which sometimes comes with heart palpitations due to fluctuating hormones.

Come On, Try It! Use this essential oil in massages and baths. It can be inhaled straight from its vial or used in a diffuser. Vanilla oil is used in fragrances, soaps, cleaning products, candles, and incense.

Calming
Vanilla Absolute Perfume

During a romantic trip to Monterey, I was suffering from PMS, which was untimely and unfortunate because it was a scenic drive on an overcast afternoon. After dodging tourist traffic and winding roads, I placed my order for a vanilla malt to go. Vanilla is one of my favorite flavors and I enjoyed its aromas in a bubble bath I took at our hotel.

I later discovered that store-bought bubble bath doesn't include vanilla absolute oil because it can contain solvents, irritates the skin, and it's expensive; synthetic vanilla is used. Vanilla extract is commonly used in a vanilla shake since vanilla absolute cannot be consumed. So I went to work and learned how to create a safe vanilla perfume to provide the benefits of a sweet-smelling shake or bath!

2 drops vanilla absolute
2 drops sandalwood essential oil
2 teaspoons jojoba oil

In a 10-ml glass roller ball container, use a glass dropper and put in both essential oils. Use a funnel to add the jojoba oil. Roll a dab on your wrists like you do for any perfume. The upside is this perfume smells sweet and earthy. The downside, though, a ⅛-ounce bottle of vanilla absolute, which contains 73 drops, cost about 70 dollars. Yes, it is pricey but making a custom-tailored scent is decadent.

(Courtesy: Plant therapy assisted me with the ratio and tools needed for making this perfume.)

SCENT-SATIONAL HEALING OILS SHORT & SWEET

✓ Put vanilla essential oil to work and use its abundance of disease-fighting antioxidants to keep your immune system healthy.

✓ Do understand the primary property of vanilla essential oil is vanillin, which scientists believe may help relax you, stave off high anxiety, stress, and uplift mood.

✓ Its eugenol and vanillin zaldehyde components are infection fighters, which are important when your body is at risk of contracting cold or flu.

✓ And note, vanilla extract—not the essential oil—is a popular flavoring that can be used in a variety of desserts from different cultures, adding more aroma and flavor.

Congratulations! You've completed my crash course on 20 essential oils (with some sidekicks) complete with their healing compounds. Now, enjoy a soak bath or perfume with vanilla essential oil, because we're taking a journey into your future. Essential oils can help you to age gracefully, decade by decade. No, not one essential oil or one compound in essential oils will stop you from growing older, but if you incorporate a variety of essential oils and aromatherapy into your life, you'll likely enjoy the journey.

PART 3

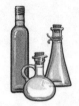

THE ESSENTIAL OILS
OF YOUTH

Aromatic Age-Fighting Oils

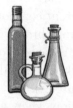

Grow old along with me!
The best is yet to be.
—ROBERT BROWNING

Using essential oils is one antidote to look young and live longer. As an aging boomer, I recall waiting for a cord of firewood to be delivered. Clad in jeans, a plaid flannel shirt, and boots, I stacked the fragrant mix of pine wood. After the work, I felt the aches and pains in my back. I whined while building a perfect fire and walking my energetic Australian shepherd in the cold air. Thirty minutes later, I did it. I escaped into Aromatherapy Land, rejuvenating my body and spirit.

I took a hot shower using a Body Bliss bath gel (from Cal-a-Vie Spa) with a mix of aromatic essential oils including amyris, lavender, neroli, petigrain, and tangerine. The mix of fragrances was invigorating and refreshing. After drying off, I dabbed a bit of lavender essential oil and jojoba oil on my dry cuticles. I put a drop of patchouli oil on my wrist to feel balanced and connected to nature. Then I cuddled up with my relaxed Australian shepherd. Living in the moment, like dogs do, I didn't feel a day over six in dog years. It's living life with passion and staying active, like I did that memorable day with the aid of oils and aromatherapy, that helps us stay vibrant and age gracefully.

OILS TO TURN BACK THE CLOCK
FOR ALL AGES

No matter what age you are (twenty or seventy), including a variety of essential oils with their potent components into your life can help you lower the risk of developing chronic ailments and age-related diseases. Aging gracefully can be done but sometimes lifestyle, genes, environment, or just the luck of the draw can hamper our best intentions to stay forever young(er).

I come from the generation when we didn't trust anyone over thirty. Fifty was considered "over the hill" aka "old." But times are changing. These days, seventy can be vibrant. And, if you lay the groundwork, such as using the right essential oils, decade after decade, you can stay forever young, as Rod Stewart's famous song title plays in my baby boomer aging mind.

From head to toe, I've provided some health issues that may affect people, decade by decade. While essential oils are not a cure-all miracle to stop the aging clock, if incorporated into the diet and lifestyle early on they very well may be one key to adding years, better health, and well-being with less aches and pains in the body and mind. Read on.

IN YOUR TWENTIES

During this decade, energizing and antiviral essential oils are in demand to stay well. Youthful, on-the-go people will often go to a walk-in clinic for urgent care for a bad cold or flu. An E.R. hospital visit is common for a serious issue, like a body injury or car accident. Women will see an ob-gyn for female issues, including pregnancy to anxiety and stress. In my twenties, I didn't think about aging because, well, at that age you feel invincible. My primary doctor was an ob-gyn. If I got a bout of the flu I would go to a clinic. I did not have health insurance.

Essential Oils for the Decade: Two of the best energizing oils for mental energy are lemon and peppermint. (Refer to the chapters on these oils and get familiarized with their components.) Two oils, chamomile and lavender, help lessen stress and anxiety, due to financial challenges, college pressures, the novelty of marriage, and starting a family.

A Scented Birthing Pool (with a Little Help of Essential Oils)

Lynda Ballard of the United Kingdom recalls the time she was pregnant and gave birth using a special method. She shares the fascinating details of an unforgettable event—and essential oils played a big role . . .

We had a birthing pool at home in the conservatory. The whole experience was magical. I can remember looking out through the glass at all the blossoms on the apple tree outside. We used clary sage and lavender in a vaporizer as a relaxant.

As the time went by, I think I became too relaxed. I can remember starting to nod off. The midwife suggested switching the oil to peppermint (a great stimulant), which helped speed things up and Lily arrived early on Sunday morning just a few hours after I had got into the pool.

IN YOUR THIRTIES

In this decade, weight loss and antistress essential oils are must-haves. It's not uncommon for men and women to seek help online through self-research and even chatting with an online doctor for advice and to find out if the health problem needs live face-to-face medical attention. Common ailments can include weight loss, depression, stress, and anxiety.

In my thirties, I was busy working as a journalist and traveling on assignments. During this decade, women often used their ob-gyn as a general health practitioner.

Essential Oils for the Decade: Good oils for stamina and brainpower are lemon and peppermint oils. Lavender and sandalwood are two picks for staying calm during ups and downs of work, with friends, and stressful family events. (Refer to the chapters on these essential oils to refresh your memory of what they do and how they can help you.)

IN YOUR FORTIES

During this decade, specific calming essential oils are desired to cope naturally with health ailments that you can control. Screenings for blood pressure, cholesterol, and diabetes are recommended to keep your numbers in check.

Essential Oils for the Decade: Excellent oils for early middle age include peppermint oil for increasing energy and pain-relieving for PMS cramps and/or aches and pains when over-exerting yourself. Antistress lavender oil is ideal for both genders in this age group.

IN YOUR FIFTIES

During this decade, it's calming and energizing essential oils that are in demand to help people to find balance. Not uncommon is a cluster of problems called metabolic syndrome—high blood pressure, high LDL "bad" cholesterol, high blood sugar—which can often be controlled with diet and lifestyle changes including essential oils.

Essential Oils for the Decade: Ginger essential oil with its gingerol compound is heart-healthy and imperative in your fifties, whether you are a man or woman. Lavender essential oil is good for coping with your aging parents and growing children, because stress often comes with the demands of being a multitask caretaker.

IN YOUR SIXTIES

By this decade, folks have an idea of what their health challenges are, and may turn to heart-healthy and immune-boosting essential oils, which are believed to lower the risk of developing heart disease and cancers. This decade can still be a healthy one if you followed a plant-based diet and healthy lifestyle in the previous years. In your sixties, having a primary healthcare doctor is commonplace. A dentist, eye doctor, and dermatologist are also common during this decade.

Essential Oils for the Decade: During your sixties, eucalyptus oil is a must-have to keep your sinuses and lungs healthy if you're bothered in colder weather or seasonal and climate changes; and it is helpful to relieve aches and pains due to keeping a move on—and doing too much, too fast. Lavender oil with its antibacterial properties can help soothe dry, irritated, and itchy skin, which sometimes happens as we age. Blending it with jojoba or coconut carrier oil is excellent for moisturizing and smoothing skin to help turn back the clock.

Anti-Aging Oil Recipe

This remedy includes two of my top 20 essential oil picks— rose and sandalwood. The other oils boast age-defying benefits, too. Neroli does, as do vetiver, borage, evening primrose, and rose hip seed oil . . .

Add the following to a small bottle:

5 drops rose essential oil
5 drops neroli essential oil
5 drops sandalwood essential oil
2 drops vetiver essential oil
1 teaspoon evening primrose oil
1 teaspoon borage oil
1 teaspoon rose hip seed oil

Apply a few drops to face and neck before each night.

(Courtesy: Annette Davis, President National Association for Holistic Aromatherapy [NAHA])

DEFY AGING WITH ESSENTIAL OILS

The thing is, we are living in the age where we live longer than ever before. Aging gracefully can make growing older and wiser easier, physically, mentally, and spiritually. I read that for the average person, if you live to sixty-five, you are likely to live another twenty years. That said, when entering your golden years, it will be more fun if you dodge diseases as the odds of developing one or more increases.

PHYSICAL: CANCER

The fact is, no one essential oil is going to be the magic cancer-fighting cure-all. Cancer can affect anyone at any age. It is the number two killer in the United States with heart disease still number one. But the chances of developing cancer increase as we age. Whether it's breast, prostate, or skin cancer, we are more at risk. But that doesn't mean we are helpless.

Diet and lifestyle are two major factors that can help us lower the risk of developing cancer, and essential oils are not to be excluded. The healing benefits that come with essential oils can help promote a healthier lifestyle because of the antioxidant-rich compounds, which can lessen stress, for one, and prevent havoc on the immune system.

"Different essential oils have been found to be effective against certain tumors in the lab," points out Kurt Schnaubelt of the Pacific Institute of Aromatherapy. "Using a wide variety of essential oils is a practice that helps to prevent the onset of cancers." The doctor points out though, that "looking for one or two active ingredients is probably not the right path." Like nutrient-dense foods, eating a wide variety of colorful fruits and vegetables is wiser than simply eating just one food to lower your risk of developing cancer.

Essential Oils That Lower Risk: Lavender essential oil contains antioxidants, including catalase, superoxide dismutase, and gluthathione, which can help fight free radical damage. It may help you to stave off aging skin and age-related cancers, such as skin cancer.

PHYSICAL: HEART DISEASE

In the twenty-first century, heart disease is a culprit but can be controlled for both men and women. My two octogenarian friends died from congestive heart failure. Like cancer, we do have some control despite genes, environmental factors, and bad luck. Eating a heart-healthy Mediterranean Diet and lifestyle, staying lean, and incorporating specific essential oils, especially ones that can lower high blood pressure, "bad" LDL cholesterol, and keep our weight in check, may help lower the risk of getting heart disease.

Essential Oils for Heart Health: Ginger essential oil is touted for its anti-inflammatory compound gingerol, which may be helpful to keep heart disease at bay. Also, lavender and peppermint oils with their calming ingredient linalool may help to soothe you. This, in return, can help keep your blood pressure numbers in check.

MENTAL: DEPRESSION

The challenge of depression is nothing new—it has affected people throughout time, but the problem is growing. Taking antidepressants is a twenty-first-century fix, but it isn't always the answer. While medication can be helpful, it often comes with side effects, such as weight gain and irregularity. Some essential oils can be helpful in the battle against depression.

Essential Oils That Boost Mood: Lavender and sandalwood all affect the olfactory system that connects the nose to the brain. Calming oils, like this duo can help balance chemicals in the brain, reducing stress and anxiety—which are often are linked to depression.

SPIRITUAL: GRIEF AND LOSS

As we age, scientists show that being isolated, lonely, and disconnected to friends and loved ones can have a negative effect on the body and aging process. When the elderly takes care of a sick spouse or family member, grief and loss can set in. These challenges can affect our well-being, whereas sleep, eating right, and quality time are often neglected. That's when essential oils can come into play.

Essential Oils That Enhance Well-Being: Chamomile essential oil can help to stave off anxiety and can promote a restful state, quieting the mind and acting as a natural sleep aid. Sleep is important for the immune system and is needed to restore and rejuvenate our bodies each day.

Aromatherapy with Essential Oils Checklist for Cancer Survivors

Here is a summary of how aromatherapy with essential oils is improving the quality of life of cancer patients—and how research is ongoing.

✓ Essential oils are used by patients with cancer mainly as supportive care for well-being.

✓ Aromatherapy is used with other complementary treatments, such as massage, as well as with standard treatments for symptom management.

✓ Research shows the sedative and stimulant effects of specific essential oils as well as the positive effects they can have on behavior and the immune system.

✓ Human clinical trials have investigated aromatherapy in the treatment of stress and anxiety in patients with critical illnesses or in other hospitalized patients. Several clinical trials involving patients with cancer have been published.

✓ Essential oils are available in the United States for inhalation and topical treatment. Topical treatments are generally used in diluted form.

(Source: National Cancer Institute)[1]

MASTERING THE ART OF AGING (AFTER THE FIRST GRAY HAIR)

As people enter their seventies and eighties and edge their way even further, other chronic and acute ailments can affect their well-being and may turn into life-threatening challenges. In the past, I had two unforgettable octogenarian friends. Geologist Jim Berkland was like a surrogate dad; my landlady, a musician-philanthropist, was my best girlfriend, a gran figure to me. Both of these people lived full and rich lives—traveling and giving to people. They both died of congestive heart failure.

The good news is, we are living longer and aging better than our parents and their parents and their parents. It may seem like a pain in the bum to start an anti-aging movement while you're tripping around the world, snowboarding at a ski resort, or working and going to college simultaneously. Who has the time for thinking about aging, right?

But when age fifty hits, you, your parents, or grandparents will be coping with the aches and pains of growing older. It's inevitable. But wait, this isn't a speech about the end being near, it's more about essential oils coming to the rescue so you can blossom for another fifty years.

At age sixty, you will most likely notice that when you get physical your stamina is less than when you were twenty. Or, if you enjoy a long day cycling, swimming, running, or working, those aches and pains may pay you a visit. It's a wake-up call to take care and essential oils can help, especially with issues like inflammation, stiffness, and skin changes and challenges, too.

Here, take a look at the most common maladies from A to Z, that can affect the elderly, which could be your parents, spouse, friends, or maybe even you.

ARTHRITIS

Stiffness in your body and joints is not uncommon as we age. However, if we follow the Mediterranean Diet and lifestyle (which includes staying active), it can help keep your body flexible. Some essential oils can boost mood and energy, making you more apt to exercise and stay fit. This can help keep your back and posture healthier, which can keep your body limber and improve your balance, making you less prone to falls.

Anti-Aging Essential Oils: Ginger essential oil with its gingerol compound is a good pain reliever and anti-inflammatory natural remedy to use, which can help lessen aches and pains. Also, eucalyptus with its eugenol compound can also reduce inflammation.

BRAINPOWER

Memory loss, dementia, and Parkinson's disease are more common in the twenty-first century as we age and live longer. Genes can play a big role; however, a healthy diet and lifestyle in conjunction with aromatherapy and essential oils may help to lower the risk of losing brainpower and keep your mind well.

Anti-Aging Essential Oils: Lavender and Rosemary essential oils work well together to boost memory and mood. In a study at the University of North Umbria, Newcastle researchers reported intriguing findings in *The International Journal of Neuroscience.* It was discovered that 144 people experienced via aromatherapy a boost in memory and alertness from the rosemary oil, and lavender provided a sense of contentment.[2]

OSTEOPOROSIS

As you age, your risk of "brittle bone" disease becomes higher. Your bones become less dense and weaker. Some bone-depleting factors include stress, inadequate peak bone mass, junk food, weak digestion, and no exercise. You have control of these culprits with the usage of essential oils and aromatherapy. Why? Some healing oils can lower stress, boost energy so you're more apt to exercise, add flavor and aroma to nutrient-dense food so your diet is healthier, and promote healthy digestion—all keys to keeping your bones stronger.

Anti-Aging Essential Oils: Ginger essential oil with anti-inflammatory coconut oil as the carrier applied to painful areas can be helpful. Also, other essentials oils, including orange, rosemary, and sage can help when used in a massage blend and/or hydrotherapy blend.

RESPIRATORY AILMENTS

Getting the flu is not fun at any age. The risk of a virus spiraling into bronchitis or even pneumonia is heightened in older people, especially if their immune system is weak. That's where immune-boosting essential oils come into play.

"The most effective oils for viral infections are those with sizable contents of cineole, mono terpene alcohol, and terpene hydrocarbons," says Kurt Schnaubelt of the Pacific Institute of Aromatherapy. He adds, "These three types of components form an effective antiviral synergy." So, it's optimal to combine essential oils in an antiviral blend as a preventative measure during flu season and if you've been exposed to someone with a flu bug.

Anti-Aging Essential Oils: Eucalyptus essential oil, which has the cinole compound, is an excellent remedy because it provides antimicrobial effects to fight against bacteria and viruses. It can be used topically or inhaled.

In terms of beauty, lavender essential oil with its antioxidants and anti-inflammation compounds can also be age-defying. Mixing ½ cup of an unscented lotion with fifteen drops of lavender oil may help reduce the appearance of fine lines.

As a baby boomer I've entered a new phase in my life. We boomers are the ones who never trusted anyone over thirty. Nowadays, I witness friends and neighbors who become the caretakers for their parents who are in their eighties. Also, my peers are now experiencing foreshadowing of their own health challenges.

So, the question is, could essential oils and aromatherapy help stall aging and lower the odds of developing health conditions? Perhaps. However, diet and lifestyle do play a significant role in staying healthier longer as we age. But if people, like me, and perhaps you, too, learn how to deal with stress, maintain a healthy weight, and use essential oils to help bolster our immune system and even act as a sunscreen we may feel and look younger.

Past lab research (done in a petri dish) suggests some essential oils provide antioxidants that protect the skin from harmful free radicals in ultraviolet rays. In fact, lavender essential oil provides 6 SPF. More research is needed on whether or not you should use the oil as a natural sunscreen.

Meanwhile, it couldn't hurt to try mixing ½ cup carrier oil, such as an unscented lotion with fifteen drops of lavender. Use with your sunscreen, like I have done, which probably has a higher SPF, such as 30.

Energizing
Essential Oil Mix Smoothie

Here is a wholesome smoothie that includes age-defying nutrients and essential oils for extra flavor and antioxidants. One day in my forties, I was at a health food store where a counter girl was whipping up my berry delight in a blender. I shook my head "no" when she asked me if I wanted special add-ins. These days, older but wiser, I make smoothies at home. They're not too sweet with syrups and not too health-oriented with chia seeds and hemp. I've got my ingredients of choice and when I savor a chilled beverage, I can rest assured that it's full of age-defying fresh organic fruits, organic milk, fortified juice with vitamins D and calcium, and antioxidant-rich dietary essential oils.

¼ cup pear, chopped
¼ cup Honeycrisp or Fuji apple, chopped
½ banana, sliced
¼ cup orange juice, fresh squeezed or fortified juice
½ cup vanilla gelato
½ cup 2 percent low-fat organic milk
1 teaspoon honey
1 teaspoon wheat germ
½ cup ice cubes
1 drop nutmeg essential oil
1 tablespoon lemon juice
1 drop cinnamon essential oil
Mint sprig (for garnish)

Blend all of the ingredients, including fruit, juices, gelato, milk, honey, wheat germ, ice, and essential oils. Pour into a glass. Garnish and serve with a straw and spoon.

Serves 1.

THE HEALING POWERS OF ESSENTIAL OILS

Welcome to the healthy, aromatic
world of essential oils!
These pictures are inspired
by the author's memories —
scents of seasons, holidays,
flavorful foods, family, and friends —
to help you discover your own
favorite essential oils.

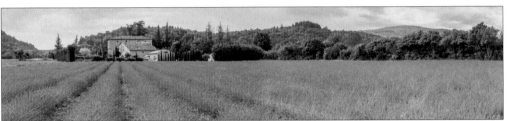

A lavender field surrounds
a French farmhouse,
lending its healing fragrance
to the countryside.
Photo by Repina Valeriya/
shutterstock.com.

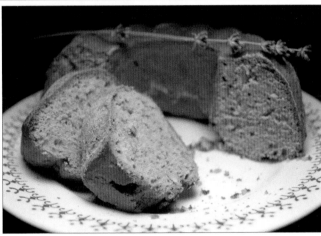

Lavender oil infused in
a Bundt cake glaze makes
this dessert extra special.
Photo by Zoltan Major/
shutterstock.com

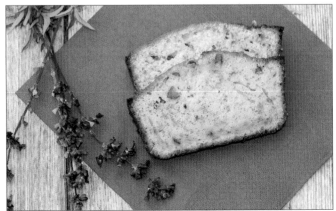

Homemade bread with a hint
of lavender essential oil has
an irresistible appeal.
Photo by naD photos/
shutterstock.com.

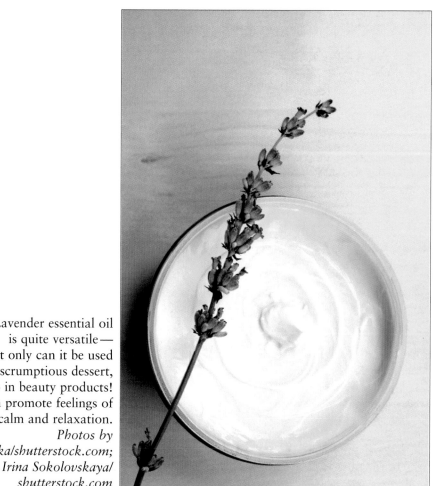

Lavender essential oil
is quite versatile —
not only can it be used
in a scrumptious dessert,
but also in beauty products!
Its scent can promote feelings of
calm and relaxation.
*Photos by
Karuka/shutterstock.com;
Irina Sokolovskaya/
shutterstock.com*

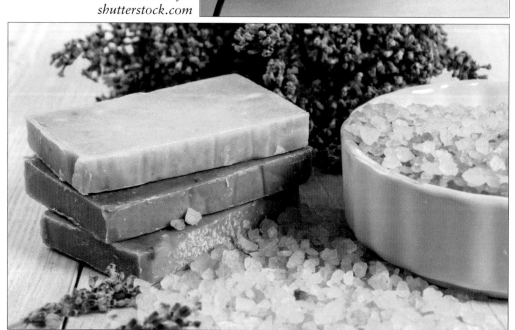

Basil essential oil can be used in delicious savory homemade dishes. It's easy and adds a little extra something.
Photo by AS Food Studio/ shutterstock.com.

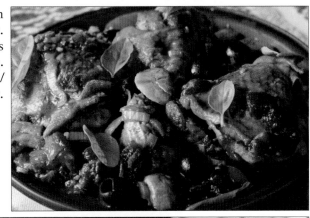

The woodsy scent of cedarwood essential oil is a perfect addition to any perfume.
Photo by Madeleine Steinbach/ shutterstock.com.

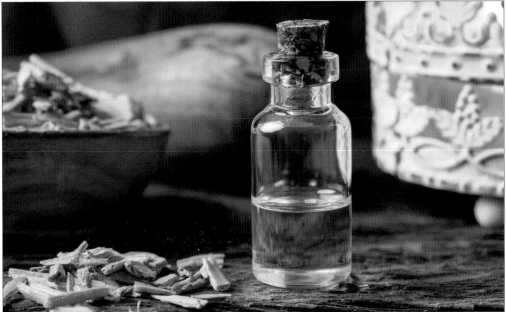

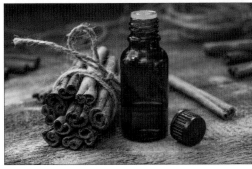

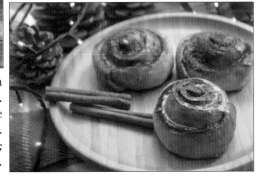

The smell of sweet and spicy cinnamon oil can ignite warm feelings. The scent is often a favorite among essential oil enthusiasts.
Photos by Bukhta Ihor/shutterstock.com; Mehriban A/shutterstock.com.

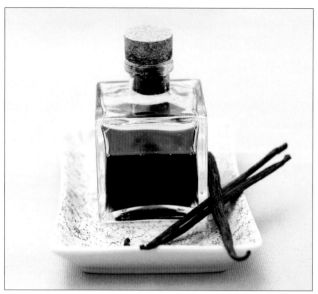

Vanilla essential oil can be used in a variety of products, including incense and potpourri. *Photos by matka_Wariatka/ shutterstock.com; Marco Mayer/shutterstock.com; Napoleonka/shutterstock.com.*

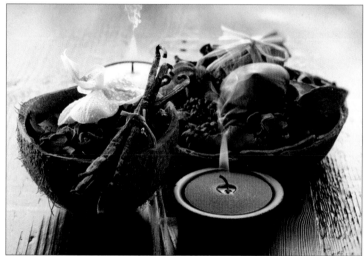

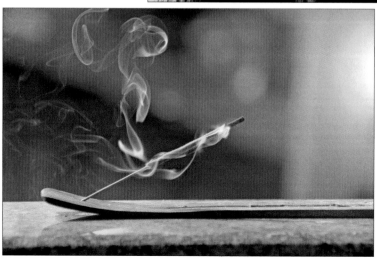

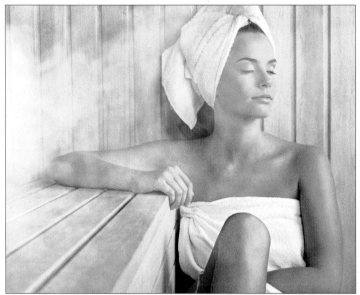

The earthy scent of eucalyptus essential oil in a spa sauna or home shower is a godsend for your health woes— and surely we all deserve such pampering.
Photo by Billion Photos/ shutterstock.com.

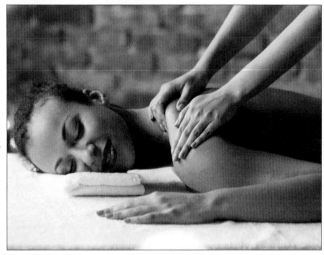

A day at the spa isn't complete without a massage. An essential oil like geranium is great as a massage oil, thanks to its healing properties.
Photo by Y Photo Studio/ shutterstock.com.

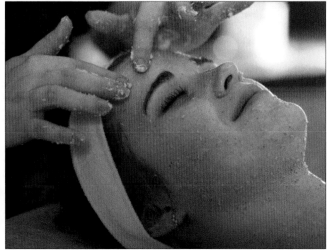

Essential oils can help exfoliate and soften your skin, making you feel radiant from morning to night.
Photo by InnerVisionPRO/ shutterstock.com.

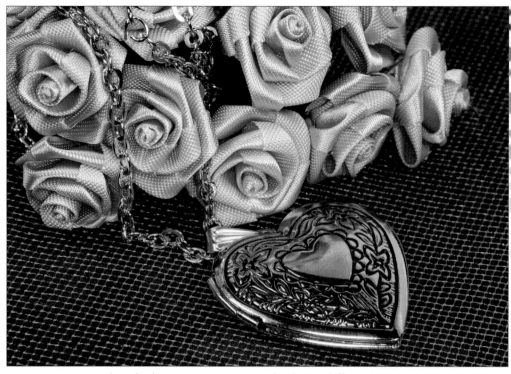

Keeping a pad soaked in geranium essential oil in a diffuser jewelry heart locket lets you keep the soothing smell of a garden with you all day long.
Photo by Scott Rothstein/shutterstock.com.

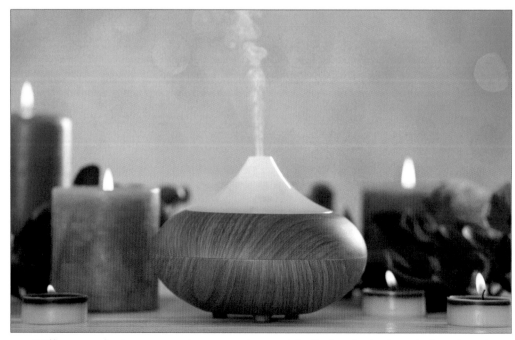

Diffusers make it easy to enjoy scented essential oils for the body, mind, and soul everywhere, from home to the office. *Photo by Africa Studio/shutterstock.com.*

Ginger essential oil releases a delightful aroma, enhancing baked goods such as gingerbread. *Photo by Margouillat Photo/ shutterstock.com.*

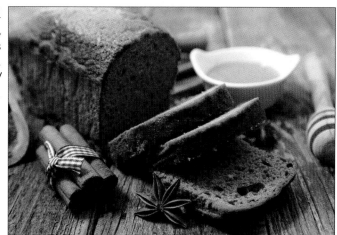

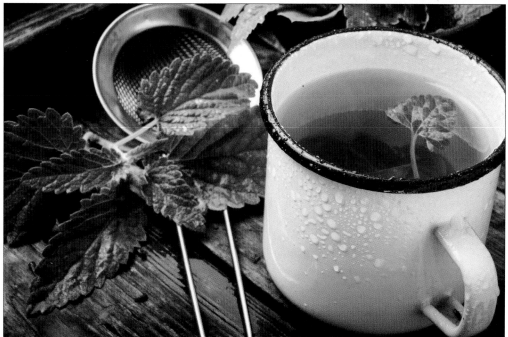

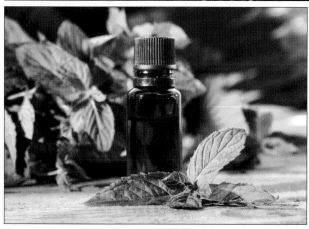

Add a drop of peppermint essential oil to a cup of tea to calm your stomach or just to get an extra energy boost. *Photos by Lunov Mykola/ shutterstock.com; Nikolay Litov/shutterstock.com.*

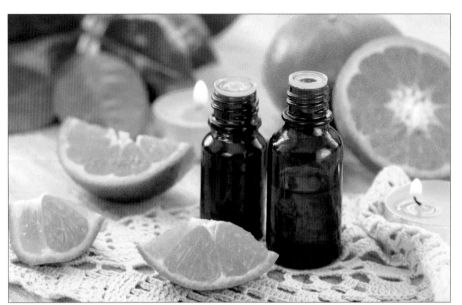

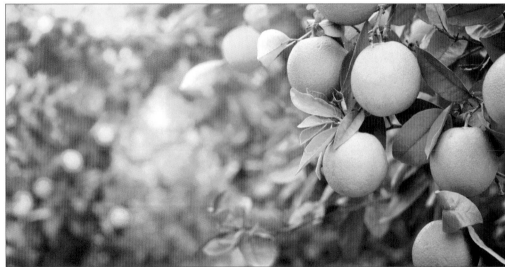

Orange essential oil's citrusy aroma is delightfully rejuvenating.
Photos by Gamzova Olga/ shutterstock.com; VAlekStudio/shutterstock.com; Billion Photos/shutterstock.com.

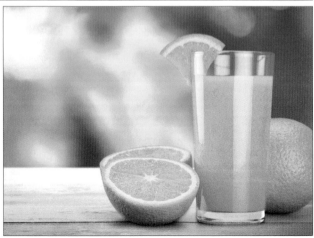

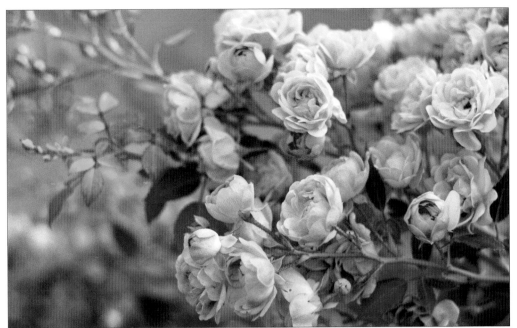

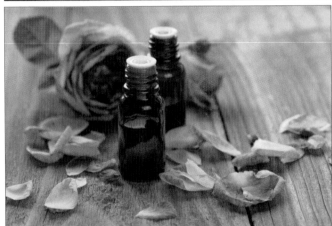

Rose oil has health benefits, such as boosting immunity and reducing cholesterol — and a pleasing fragrance, too! *Photos by Dmitrij Yakovets/ shutterstock.com; Epitavi/shutterstock.com.*

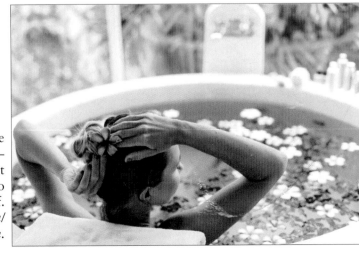

Rose oil can also be used in your bath — a luxurious delight when you want to treat yourself. *Photo by Alena Ozerova/ shutterstock.com.*

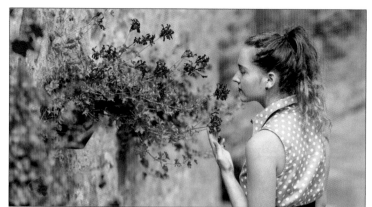

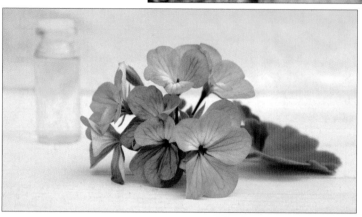

Jasmine essential oil, like geranium essential oil, has a floral fragrance that is inviting and has been found to enhance confidence and well-being. *Photos by Andriy Blokhin/ shutterstock.com; Oxik/shutterstock.com; GCapture/shutterstock.com; Pond's Saksit/shutterstock.com.*

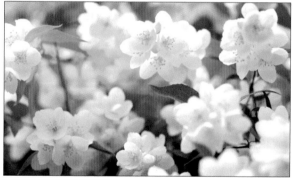

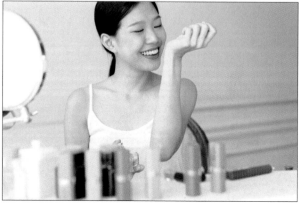

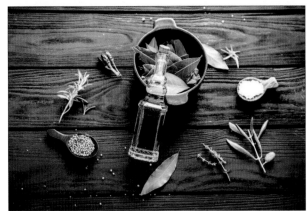

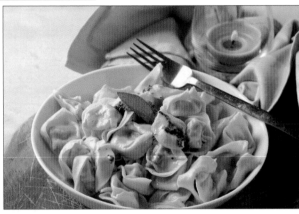

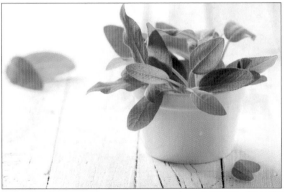

Olive oil, as a carrier oil, mixed with herbal essential oils like sage, can add irresistible aroma and flavor to a pasta dish. *Photos by Mythja/shutterstock.com; Francesco83/shutterstock.com; Oxana Denezhkina/shutterstock.com; Dusan Zidar/shutterstock.com.*

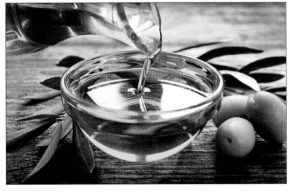

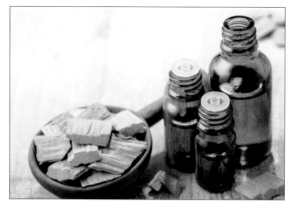

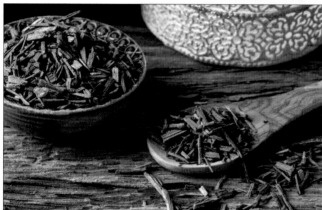

Sandalwood essential oil provides a soothing aroma. Use sandalwood incense to unwind before bed, or dab some sandalwood essential oil on your wrist to stay calm throughout the day.
Photos by AmyLv/ shutterstock.com; Madeleine Steinbach/ shutterstock.com; Kong Act/shutterstock.com; New Africa/shutterstock.com.

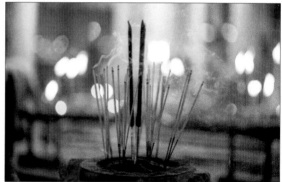

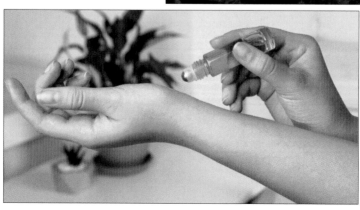

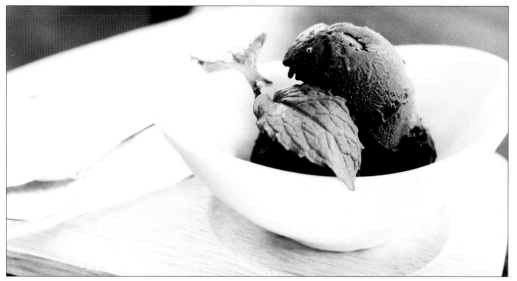

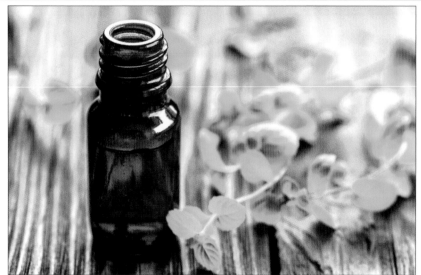

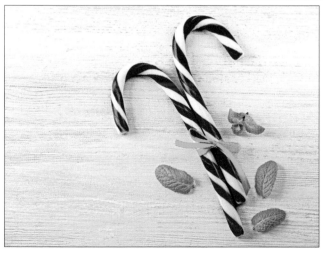

Spearmint is often used in candies and can also flavor ice cream for a decadent treat.
Photos by Wutzkohphoto/ shutterstock.com; Sea Wave/shutterstock.com; Africa Studio/shutterstock.com.

Culinary essential oils can take a dish to the next level. Basil essential oil is a welcome addition to any homemade tomato sauce. *Photos by Patricia Chumillas/shutterstock.com; Mzuzka/shutterstock.com.*

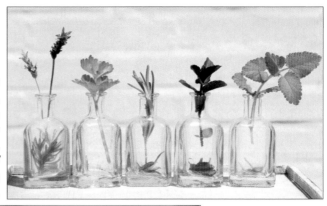

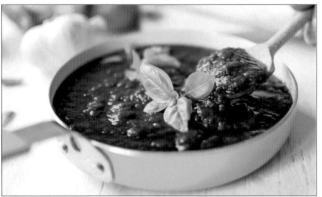

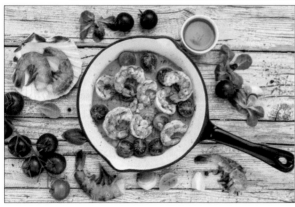

Rosemary essential oil can make a Mediterranean dish even more flavorful. *Photos by iMarzi/shutterstock.com; Dani Vincek/shutterstock.com.*

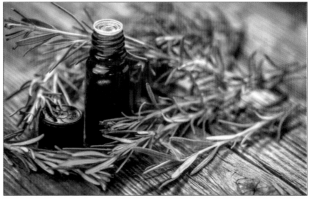

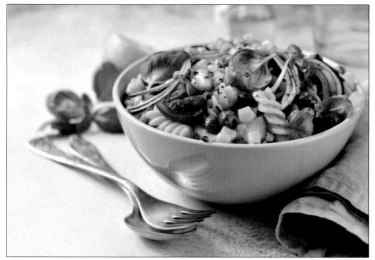

Pasta salad with a citrus twist of essential oil is a sure hit for a cooling summer lunch. *Photos by Liliya Kandrashevich/ shutterstock.com; IgorZh/ shutterstock.com; Bowonpat Sakaew/ shutterstock.com.*

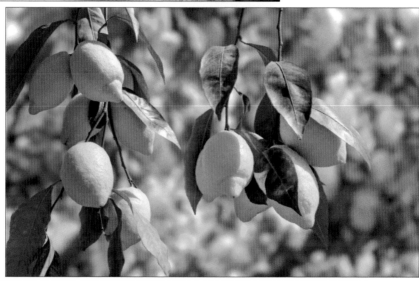

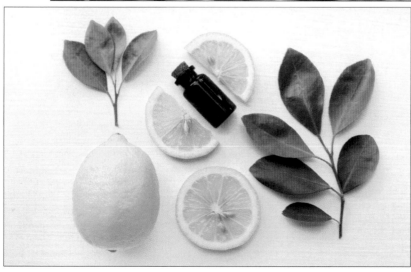

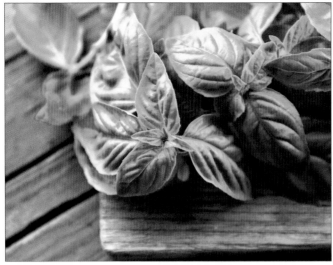

A bowl of hot chicken soup with a hint of basil essential oil is perfect when you're feeling under the weather. The oil's bacteria-fighting compounds will help you feel better.
Photos by Africa Studio/ shutterstock.com; Andrey Starostin/ shutterstock.com.

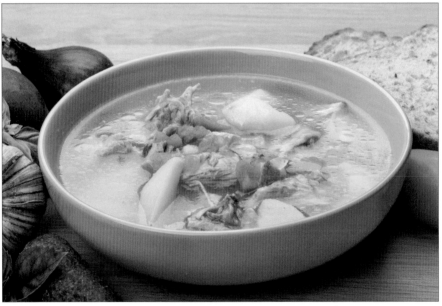

Essential oils provide numerous health benefits and promote soothing relaxation. Incorporate them into your lifestyle and reap the rewards!
Photo by Madeleine Steinbach/ shutterstock.com.

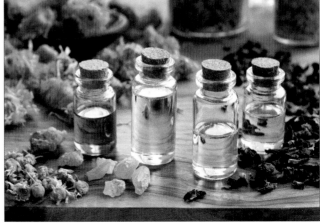

So yes, we can age gracefully. Essential oils can play a role in living a less stressful life. They can help you to relax and rejuventate your body, mind, and spirit each and every day. Next up I'm going to show you exactly how using the right essential oils can help you maintain your optimum body weight—a key to staying healthier. Discover how slimming essential oils can be your best friend for life.

SCENT-SATIONAL HEALING OILS SHORT & SWEET

✓ Did you know you can look and feel younger when using essential oils because they can refuel your mind, body, and spirit by helping you to relax and rejuvenate yourself.

✓ Antioxidant-rich essential oils may also help lower your risk of developing heart disease and cancer.

✓ Using different essential oils and learning to put them to work in a variety of methods, from inhaling, topically, and consuming will help you to stay younger, feel younger.

The Slimming Essentials

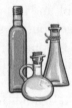

*Behave so the aroma of your actions may enhance
the general sweetness of the atmosphere.*
—HENRY DAVID THOREAU

During the holidays and celebrations year-round, the scent of essential oils can help curb your appetite while temptation to overindulge in festive foods and beverages can pack unwanted pounds. One afternoon while shopping at our local grocery store, I stopped at the Starbucks kiosk. I sniffed the smell of vanilla petit scones made with vanilla extract, remembering it contains the same compounds as the essential oil. Inhaling the fragrance of sweet vanilla gave me a food fix, and just like cuddling a warm puppy, you don't always take one home.

After the store run, I swam at the resort swimming pool. In the locker room I took a dip in the hot tub. It was full of well-groomed, middle-aged women on vacation. The words "You're so skinny!" echoed while I listened to the antics of their failing yo-yo diets and how they felt they resembled a group of food-loving plump penguins.

"I look but don't touch," I whispered when the tub bubbles stopped. But I fessed up. "I can gain a muffin top if I eat too much of something I bake."

Then, I turn to a plant-based, aromatic semi-fast to dump unwanted pounds. Dead silence. I envisioned the women inhaling essential oils and liking the effortless way to slim down and shape up.

THE SCIENCE BEHIND SKINNY SCENTS

My tip to the tourists wasn't too far-fetched. Past research at Duke Medical Center actually showed dieters used food-scented flavor enhancers and sprays to satisfy their food cravings instead of eating fattening fare. Using aroma to curb one's appetite seems to work, and more studies are proving it works wonders for weight loss because it counteracts mindless overeating.

Stress eating is also a big problem for people of all ages and both genders. Turning to antistress and anti-anxiety essential oils, such as chamomile and lavender, may help to calm the nervous system and help people chill instead of reaching for food when they are not hungry but stressed out. We often reach for comfort foods to alleviate stress, but then after overindulging in unhealthy foods, such as potato chips or packaged pastries, we feel more stressed because we know it's empty nutrition and it can pack on more unwanted pounds, creating a vicious cycle.

BEST SLIMMING OILS

Take a look at my favorite tried-and-true essential oils from A to Z that may be your best friends when you are determined to shed unwanted pounds and body fat. Some of these oils are gleaned from my top 20 picks, but I also share other oils that can be even more useful for slimming down, and shaping up. These slimming oils can be used for all seasons, from getting extra fall energy, losing winter weight gain, as a springtime detox, and for a summer pounds-off program.

CINNAMON OIL

Ah, spicy cinnamon aroma leads the pack of slimming essential oils. Medical researchers believe this oil, which can be used topically, inhaled, and ingested, may help steady the sugar levels in your body. Steady blood sugar numbers will stabilize your mood and energy.

Using cinnamon essential oil in any form is also believed to lessen food cravings for sugary foods, which are called "trigger foods"— culprits like empty nutrition cookies and candy that can often trigger you to eat one after the other, right into the "I ate the whole thing" dilemma.

The Slim Down Method: Add 1 drop of cinnamon oil to a fresh fruit salad like Meg Ryan's character puts together in the film *City of Angels*. Her sense of smell is heightened as she puts together a fruit bowl in the morning, savoring all of the earthy scents, including lemon. Or blend up a smoothie full of fruit, yogurt, a bit of raw honey mixed with a drop of cinnamon oil for extra savory flavor.

Cinnamon leaf oil contains a component that may change our neurosensory perceptions and change how we taste and smell food. This, in turn, may actually stave off food cravings and curb overeating. In other words, take time to smell the food and enjoy each and every bite rather than wolfing down the garden without enjoying the beauty of it.

GINGER OIL

Here is another spicy oil, like cinnamon oil, which may lower sugar cravings. The active compounds in ginger are gingerols, which research suggests makes ginger oil a cortisol reducer (a hormone that can contribute to belly body fat).

Slim Down Scent Method: You can put one drop in eight ounces of hot chamomile tea (for a calming effect) and a fresh mint sprig for flavor or a slice of orange. The Food and Drug Administration notes ginger essential oil is safe to ingest, but use therapeutic grade oil. Or simply whiff the scent straight from a vial of the oil.

GRAPEFRUIT OIL

This citrus essential oil, much like the fruit, is known for its fat-burning perks. I recall using the low-calorie grapefruit diet, popular in the twentieth century. It was a quickie diet including cottage cheese, salad, and black coffee. The grapefruit was believed to be fat-burning and got credit with people, like me, who want to lose unwanted weight fast. Aromatherapists believe grapefruit oil aids your body to break down fat. Interestingly, grapefruit oil is one ingredient included in anti-cellulite creams.

Also, grapefruit oil comes from the grapefruit peel and contains the compound D-limonene; it may help rev up your metabolism aka calorie-burning power. This oil may act as a diuretic like water-rich fruits and vegetables, which can help you lose water weight as a jump-start incentive to dump unwanted pounds.

Dr. Ann Louise Gittleman touts grapefruit essential oil as a tool for weight loss. She also recommends two other essential oils for fat loss, lemongrass and cypress.

Slim Down Scent Method: Use grapefruit oil solo or combined with a carrier oil, such as jojoba oil for a daily massage by applying to your belly, upper thighs, and buttocks.

Weight Loss Recipe

Add the following to a small bottle:

1 teaspoon plus 30 drops grapefruit essential oil
1 teaspoon plus 30 drops lemon essential oil
30 drops cardamom essential oil
30 drops peppermint oil
30 drops cinnamon oil

To help control hunger pangs or cravings for junk food, drink a glass of lemon water, then inhale essential oil blend until the hunger/cravings pass. Place a couple of drops onto a tissue or cotton pad. **Caution:** Avoid contact with eyes and mucous membranes. Keep out of reach of children and pets.

(Courtesy: Annette Davis, President National Association for Holistic Aromatherapy [NAHA])

JASMINE OIL

If you're coping with weight issues compounded by stress at home or the workplace—or both—it's time to turn to an oil that can relax you. Often anxiety and stress can come with depression, but jasmine is believed to uplift your spirits. And if you're feeling better about yourself, you are less apt to reach for unhealthy foods as a temporary fix for your mood.

Slim Down Scent Method: Put one or two drops of jasmine oil on a cotton ball and inhale the aroma. Repeat as necessary.

LAVENDER OIL

Research shows essential lavender oil may not only lower stress levels but it could also suppress the desire to give into emotional eating. Lavender oil is also known to lower cortisol levels, the stress hormone that makes your body hold on to stubborn body fat—especially around your belly. The fragrance enters the amygdala or the brain's center of emotions, which may lessen anxiety and stress—the two emotions that trigger mindless eating.

Slim Down Scent Method: Rub two drops of lavender oil diluted with two drops of jojoba or almond oil on your wrists. Or you can also take a whiff of the oil straight from a small bottle or vial.

LEMON OIL

This citrusy fresh essential oil contains the medicinal compound limonene, which is believed to be a "fat dissolver" or it can help eliminate unwanted body fat. Lemons and lemon oil are known detoxifiers that can get rid of toxins in the body that can be stored as fat cells, dietitians say.

Slim Down Scent Method: Add one drop of lemon essential oil into a glass of cold water or hot water. Add a bit of honey and a sprig of mint.

PEPPERMINT OIL

It's the menthol in peppermint essential oil that can affect neurosensory preconceptions to switch up on how we taste and smell food. This, in turn, can help lower cravings for sugary or high fat foods after eating healthful fare, especially during the holiday season, a time when festive food—think turkey stuffing, gravy, pie—is a big temptation to resist.

Slim Down Scent Method: Add one to two drops of peppermint oil to a glass of hot water. Try this remedy before dinner to help curb your appetite.

ROSEMARY OIL

Extracted from rosemary sprigs through steam distillation, this slimming essential oil can be another dieter's best friend. Like lavender, it may have the power to fight cortisol, the stress hormone, which can lead to emotional eating and weight gain around the belly.

Slim Down Scent Method: Take a few whiffs of rosemary oil from the bottle or vial. Repeat as needed.

SANDALWOOD OIL

Like chamomile and lavender oils, this oil can help provide you with a calming effect. It is believed to have a therapeutic effect on the limbic system of the brain (remember, it's the part that controls emotions and hunger). Incorporating this oil into your life may help you to feel more grounded, whereby overeating or eating the foods without nutritional value will be history.

Slim Down Scent Method: Take a whiff or two straight from the small bottle of sandalwood essential oil and/or dab an undiluted drop on your wrist. Also, try putting a few drops on a pad and putting it inside a jewelry diffuser necklace.

VANILLA

Sniffing the right aroma, like I told the group of women in the hot tub, can trick your brain into thinking you're full and help to reduce your appetite. Researchers at the Smell and Taste Treatment and Research Foundation in Chicago, Illinois, discovered more than three thousand people between the ages of eighteen and sixty-four who smelled peppermint essential oil lost weight. The people were given inhalers of aromatic ingredients such as bananas, green apples, and peppermint. The findings: In a six-month period, the average pounds dropped by individuals was close to five pounds each month. This, in result, was enough evidence to claim that aroma may help in losing weight.[1]

Slim Down Scent Method: Try a vanilla oil aromatic massage or bath. Light a vanilla-scented essential oil–infused candle. Use vanilla oil in a diffuser or vaporizer. Put one or two drops of the oil on a handkerchief and sniff.

Pare Pounds with Massage

We know massages can help you to destress, loosen up tight muscles like hydrotherapy or swimming. Some essential oils, applied directly to the skin, may also help your body to lose weight. "In some cases, massage and body oil with the following ingredients can be of help," says Monika Haas, managing director of the Pacific Institute of Aromatherapy.

95 mL coconut oil
10 drops grapefruit essential oil
10 drops cypress essential oil

10 drops lemon essential oil
5 drops fennel essential oil

Use this formula like other massage oil mixtures. You can rub it into your skin or have someone else do it. Rinse after.

Haas added another weight loss trick that may help. Or not. In France, 1 drop of lavender essential oil is ingested every two hours. Evidently, it may balance the insulin production in the body and counteract sugar cravings. Use food grade oil only and I recommend diluting it with a glass of water or 1 teaspoon of honey.

EMOTIONAL EATING? ESSENTIAL OILS 9-1-1!

My former easygoing neighbor, a young woman, preparing for her wedding, felt overwhelmed with the happy but stressful event. When her fiancé was at work, she'd take out pastries hidden in a bread box. She told me wolfing down six sweet rolls would help calm her jittery nerves, but admits she didn't even enjoy the forbidden food. A teenager late at night felt overwhelmed about not fitting in at her new school. To cope, she would binge on cookies to fill the void and feel happier (I was that girl). A man (actually, an ex-boyfriend of mine) faced politics at a high-stress job. During lunch and after work, he would turn to fast food to feel better, but the weight gain made him feel worse.

What do these three have in common? They turn to unhealthy food to mask the problem that is eating away at their emotions. Medical researchers and experts who deal with people's eating disorders believe a mixed bag of feelings, including anger, anxiety guilt, and sadness can trigger overeating.

A study at Kagoshima University in Japan, published in *Frontiers in Behavioral Neuroscience*, shows that inhaling linalool may be helpful in behavioral modification. This compound found in both lavender and peppermint essential oils, and others, report the researchers, can cause calming effects, which can help to reduce stress and anxiety. More research is needed, since this was a lab study with rodents, but the results show promise.[2]

So if people sniff the right essential oil, mindless eating may not occur. At home, you could put a drop of lavender or peppermint essential oil into a glass of water or cup of tea, sip and feel less anxious and not be tempted to fill up those negative emotions with food. Or consider going to the gym and inhaling a scent such as patchouli or sandalwood to help feel more centered and in control.

Essential oils and aromatherapy can help people relax, destress, and fight anxiety. By doing this, it makes it easier to begin mindful eating. You will only eat when hungry and in order to nourish your body. The bottom line: Essential oils can be a tool in curbing the appetite, boosting mood, reducing stress, depression, and anxiety.

LOSE UP TO SEVEN POUNDS ON A WEEKEND AROMATHERAPY DIET

Staying lean 365 days a year would be wonderful but it's not realistic. Sometimes, we end up overindulging or are less active, and pounds can pile on, one by one. I'm not going to lie. Sometimes I do give in to temptation when testing recipes, and those familiar five pesky pounds, especially when wearing my favorite jeans, haunt me. I can feel the pudge around my waist. But essential oils come to the rescue.

Welcome to a satisfying jump-start plant-based semi-fast complete with essential oils and aromatherapy. This two-day diet is easiest to follow on a weekend at home so you can have control of what you eat and the environment you create. You can use it periodically, but do not use it back-to-back or on a weekly basis.

It's a nice detox diet plan to follow for each season: fall for boosting your immune system; winter to lose pounds after indulging in holiday fare; spring to detox; and summer to energize. It's best to use it for two days to kick your calorie-burning power up a notch or two. Think of it as a fresh start, especially after eating too much, or before a special event so you can fit into that favorite dress or skinny jeans without a struggle.

This diet plan is a cleansing, detoxing spin-off of the infinite number of mini-fasts I've developed with the help of a variety of nutritionists. What I love about this two-day mini-fast is that it's all fresh food–flavored combined with metabolism-boosting essential oils, aromas, and extra taste. This way you're getting healthful plant-based foods from the Oldways Mediterranean pyramid and extra taste so you will not feel deprived.

THE ESSENTIAL OILS DIET FEEL-GOOD RULES—JUST FOR YOU!

✓ Sniff for happiness after 7 P.M. instead of stress snacking . . . take an aromatic bath or shower using essential oils to calm you.

✓ If your stomach growls or you want to munch on junk food, drink bottled water or hot/iced tea spiked with a drop of mint oil to curb your cravings.

✓ Before starting this mini-semi-fast, consult with your health practitioner and find out if it's safe for you since every individual is different. No one weight loss diet fits all.

✓ Do not use this mini-fast if you're pregnant, nursing, or have diabetes.

✓ Drink six to eight (eight-ounce) glasses of water each day to fill you up, keep you regular and hydrated.

✓ Do not go below one thousand calories. Remember, this is a jump-start two-day semi-fast and not meant to be any longer.

✓ Pamper You! Get an aromatic massage; use a mist vaporizer; wear aromatic jewelry.

✓ Bottom line: Treat your body and spirit like royalty with the gift of essential oils and aromatherapy instead of overindulging in unhealthy foods.

✓ Try yoga, walking on a treadmill, or swimming—all of these help you to be focused, calm, and more fit.

Day 1

Pre-Breakfast:
Lemon Water (use 1 drop of lemon essential oil in 8 ounces of spring, filtered, or bottled water)

Breakfast:
Fresh fruit; 2 eggs, scrambled or hard boiled

Snack:
Raw vegetables and herbal tea

Lunch:
Spinach salad with cruciferous vegetables; tomatoes with oil and vinegar dressing; 1 toothpick drop of lemon essential oil; tea

Dinner:
4 ounces brown rice with toothpick amount of basil essential oil diluted with 1 teaspoon olive oil; 1 cup cruciferous vegetables

Snack:
1 cup fresh berries or melon

Day 2

Pre-Breakfast:
Double Mint-Flavored Water (use 1 drop of lemon essential oil diluted with 2 teaspoons of honey in 12 ounces of spring, filtered, or bottled water)

Breakfast:
¾ cup oatmeal with ½ cup low-fat organic milk; ½ grapefruit with droplet of cinnamon essential oil; 1 cup quality coffee or green tea

Lunch:
1 cup whole grain pasta mixed with ½ cup each sliced tomatoes and broccoli. Top with 1 teaspoon olive oil and 1 toothpick drop of rosemary essential oil; 1 orange

Snack:
1 apple

Dinner:
4 ounces chicken breast or turkey; 1 cup kale and cabbage mixed with olive oil, red wine vinegar; 1 toothpick drop of rosemary essential oil

Snack:

1 cup grapes, mix green and purple; 1 cup tea with 1 toothpick drop lemon or cinnamon essential oil diluted with 1 teaspoon of honey

Pound-Paring Grapefruit Salad With Lemon Oil Mint Dressing

❖ ❖ ❖

1 medium beet, cooked, diced
2 green onions (white part) sliced thin
1 pound crab meat (picked over) or shrimp, cooked
2 cups red or regular grapefruit, sectioned
2 cups fennel bulb or celery, sliced thin
1 small head red leaf or Bibb lettuce, chopped
1 head of Belgian endive, sliced thin or curly endive,
*   chopped*
2 cups dandelion or watercress, chopped
1 cup radicchio or red cabbage, shredded
1 cup blueberries or strawberries

In a large shallow serving bowl, combine beet, onions, shellfish, grapefruit, lettuce, endive, watercress, cabbage, and berries. Pour dressing over and toss gently. Keep refrigerated until ready to serve. Garnish with sprigs of fresh mint.

Serves 4 to 6.

(Courtesy: *Cooking with California Olive Oil: Popular Recipes*, Gemma Sanita Sciabica)

LEMON OIL MINT DRESSING

¼ cup red grapefruit juice, fresh or store-bought
⅓ cup light olive oil
¼ cup raw honey
1 drop lemon essential oil
¼ cup fresh mint
Ground pepper and sea salt to taste

In a small bowl whisk juice, olive oil, honey, lemon oil, mint, and spices. Cover and chill in the refrigerator.

Now that you're in the loop of how to utilize essential oils and aromatherapy to watch your weight, it's time to take our oils and scents to another place. Yes, these essential oils can do much more than take off body fat and pounds. My favorite essential oils can help you to cope with acute or chronic ailments that affect you. Yes, ancient oils can help you heal present-day health ailments. Read on—to discover these amazing folk remedies.

SCENT-SATIONAL HEALING OILS SHORT & SWEET

✓ Using essential oils is the key to stoking your metabolism (calorie-burning power) and keeping lean.
✓ Smelling oils and fragrant foods will lessen cravings for unhealthy fare to help fill you up in your mind and not out in your body.
✓ Adding a balance of food-grade essential oils paired with the carrier oil olive oil will help you feel satiated . . .
✓ Flavoring foods with a bit of essential oils is a good slimming substitute for fats, salt, and sugar.
✓ Stay true to the Mediterranean Diet and essential oils to maintain good heart health and a healthy weight.

PART 4

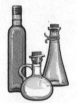

HOME REMEDIES

Home Cures from Your Kitchen

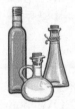

No disease that can be treated by diet should be treated with any other means.
—MAIMONIDES

In early spring, one year I traveled through a thriller film–like whiteout snowstorm to Reno for a book signing. An aromatic pendant necklace with a potent smelling patchouli oil pad helped me chill, but I craved an anti-anxiety essential oil arsenal. I was coping with my dog who just had his canine flu shot, and a cranky sibling who wanted to be anywhere but on the ice rink roads. Worse, while the new book had sold out before my arrival, the store wasn't busy and I was not Stephen King, but the Misery day felt nightmarish.

Despite lack of preparedness, except for the aromatic jewelry, we survived the one-hundred-mile trek. Once home I lit a lavender-scented candle and took a long shower, using a body gel with a mix of essential oils. After the bathroom escape, I sipped a large cup of chamomile tea with a drop of cinnamon oil. I was warm, cozy, and in my comfort zone in a homemade scented heaven to calm the stressful day of travel and chaos.

Do-it-yourself home cures are a growing trend in the twenty-first century. People of all ages are seeking essential oils to use solo or in a blend to help take care of a galling health ailment.

In an A-to-Z order, you'll find forty-five plus extra essential oil treatments to try for curing a problem, like our mothers and grand-mothers would do. It can save you from a doctor's visit and give you a sense of control, too. I include my top 20 essential oils, but also toss in a few other essential oils for a solo remedy or blend to provide effec-tive do-it-yourself home care.

If you're wondering about what brands to use, try the well-known names first, as I have done, to gain trust and feel confident and com-fortable with each essential oil and aromatherapy accessory. These in-clude Aura Cacia, doTerra, NOWFoods, Plant Therapy, and Young Living, which are available from essential oil companies, health foods stores, drugstores, and online. (Check out the Essential Oils Re-sources located in the end of this book for contact information.)

Also, I provide different ways on how to use essential oils and aro-matherapy for each home cure. Often, I will note which compounds make the oil do its job; you can find additional details in previous chapters on each essential oil. And, keep in mind, these single essen-tial oils and/or blends also can be used for beauty and the household, which follow home remedies, showing you that essential oils are multi-purpose. So when you discover your favorites, you'll be surprised that you can use them in so many different ways. These essential oil reme-dies are my favorite ones.

You'll also discover some of these remedies are backed up by med-ical studies, personal stories, and folklore. I use a dash of anecdotes from people I've known, along with words of wisdom gleaned from aromatherapists and naturopaths. Also I went to folks from big and small essential oil and aromatherapy companies who understand the powers of oils and scents and are eager to share their findings. At the end of this section, enjoy the essential oils comprehensive chart shared by NOWFoods, which will show you the best blends and how they can help you.

ESSENTIAL REMEDY #1: ACNE—BANISH BLEMISHES! BLOT WITH TEA TREE.

Simply put, acne is inflamed sebaceous glands in the skin and it can include pimples, blackheads, and whiteheads. Blame the common condition on hormones, pre-menstrual syndrome, your parents, stress, and even the weather! I did cope with acne as a teen. Then, in my thirties when traveling to humid Hawaii, I ended up with blotchy red spots on my face. The technical term of breakouts from warm weather is "tropical acne." Since then I have discovered an essential oil fix to help clear up my face if I travel to a warm region and get a rash of blemishes.

What Scent-sational Oil Rx to Use: Combine ½ cup water, 2 tablespoons apple cider vinegar with 4 drops of tea tree essential oil. Use a cotton ball and apply mixture on blemishes. Wipe mixture with water immediately. Repeat 2 to 3 times daily.

Why You'll Essentially Feel Fine: Tea tree oil contains anti-inflammatory and antibacterial compounds. Both of these can help dry up blemishes as does vinegar, which also provides the same benefits. Combining the apple cider vinegar with tea tree oil can speed up healing time. One Southern California millennial proved it. While swimming laps at the resort pool, we talked about her trip to Queensland, Australia.

She told me, "I got terrible breakouts when I was there."

She blamed it mostly on the humid air. Tea tree essential oil came to her rescue. She used the oil undiluted, and her sensitive skin, she told me, was irritated. Once she diluted it with vinegar and water the results were better.

ESSENTIAL REMEDY #2: ANXIETY—SNIFF IT! AH, THE TAO OF SANDALWOOD.

Feeling on edge? You're hardly alone. According to the Anxiety and Depression Association of America, anxiety disorder is the most common mental illness in the United States, affecting forty million adults age eighteen and older. Blame it on genetics, out-of-whack brain chemicals, personality, and life events. High anxiety can come with a variety of symptoms. It is often linked to stress and poor coping skills. Worrying about "what if" instead of living in the now can make anxiety soar. If your muscles feel tight, you have racing thoughts, your heart pounds fast, and you don't feel grounded, you're probably anxious.

What Scent-sational Oil Rx to Use: Put a few drops of a calming essential oil, such as sandalwood, on a pad and insert it in an aromatherapy diffuser necklace or put a drop or two on your wrist. Inhale a few times. Repeat as needed.

Why You'll Essentially Feel Fine: Earthy essential oils like woodsy sandalwood boast those calming sesquiterpenes that affect the nervous system so you can relax. (Go back to the chapter on sandalwood.) The beauty of wearing a diffuser necklace is that whether you're anxious at home or elsewhere, you have the luxury of taking a whiff of a natural scent that can help soothe your nerves. Also, taking an aromatherapy bath or getting a spa massage can calm the nervous system, but they're not as convenient.

I remember wearing a stainless steel aromatic diffuser necklace. When I walked my late Brittany through a woodsy trail, it was necessary for me to stay calm and maintain assertive energy in case we faced any challenges, such as coyotes, cougars, or bears. By inhaling sandalwood oil, it helped me maintain my alpha position and stay calm to enjoy our nature walks in all four seasons.

ESSENTIAL REMEDY #3: ASTHMA ATTACK—HARNESS YOUR BREATHING POWER! INHALE EUCALYPTUS.

Asthma is a chronic disease that can inflame the walls of passageways that supply air to the lungs. Inflamed airways aggravated by stress or toxins can cause difficulty breathing, including coughing and wheezing. Nobody is immune. A next-door neighbor has chronic asthma and uses an inhaler. My friend's wife, at forty-eight, died from an acute asthma attack. I've watched films with kids who have asthma and during stressful events they need an inhaler. If you have asthma under control with conventional medicine but want extra precautionary measures, essential oils may be included in your medicinal oils for asthma attacks.

What Scent-sational Oil Rx to Use: Apply 2 drops of eucalyptus oil to 1 cup of steaming hot water. Inhale the steam. Or put 1 or 2 drops of oil on a handkerchief or cotton ball and sniff. Repeat as needed.

Why You'll Essentially Feel Fine: If you have smelled the distinct, strong aroma of eucalyptus you know it can help clear airways. Thanks to the eucalyptol in eucalyptus essential oil, it has the ability to allow you to breathe easier, stay calmer, and help prevent an asthma attack.

ESSENTIAL REMEDY #4: ATHLETE'S FOOT—STOP THE ITCH QUICK! USE PEPPERMINT POWER.

Welcome to a common fungal skin infection that often is found between the toes and can spread on the feet. It occurs when people have sweaty feet and wear shoes that are not a good fit. Athlete's foot is contagious. You can contract it easily, and often by walking barefoot in a gym or swimming pool locker room area. The end result: A rash and itchy and burning feet.

What Scent-sational Oil Rx to Use: Use a topical cream. In a small jar blend ½ cup of all-natural unscented lotion. Add 3 drops of an antifungal peppermint essential oil. You can use an aromatherapy soap that contains peppermint oil. Use the lotion or soap twice per day until healed.

Why You'll Essentially Feel Fine: Peppermint oil helps cure the itch and burn with its antifungal and anti-inflammatory compounds. As a teen I recall my sister had bouts of athlete's foot, which seemed to happen during swim club season. She used this medicinal over-the-counter cream that smelled like rotten eggs. Since I have a strong sense of smell, a more fragrant cure would have been welcomed and wouldn't have resulted in the sibling bickering that her more pungent solution caused.

ESSENTIAL REMEDY #5: BOILS—HEAL THE BUMP(S)! GO VANILLA.

A swollen red bump filled with pus under your skin could potentially be a boil. A sore like this can cause inflammation or an infection of the hair follicles, often caused by staphylococcus. If the boil is small, self-care with a compress and essential oil can be all that is needed without a visit to a doctor.

What Scent-sational Oil Rx to Use: Put 3 to 5 drops of vanilla essential oil into ½ cup water. Dab a clean washcloth into the oil and water potion and press the cloth onto the boil for 15 minutes. Repeat twice a day.

Why You'll Essentially Feel Fine: Amazingly, sweet-smelling vanilla essential oil contains antibacterial compounds, including eugenol and vanillin hydroxybenzaldehyde. This powerful pair can fight bacteria and fight infection. A friend of mine had a tiny boil on his chin underneath a beard. He resisted home remedies, like this one, and ended up going to a dermatologist to have it removed. Perhaps the vanilla essential oil treatment could have saved him a doctor's visit.

ESSENTIAL REMEDY #6: BRUISES—REV UP HEALING! ROSEMARY RECOVERY.

A bruise is an injury to the skin that often shows discoloration. Blood from damaged blood cells underneath the skin end up as a black and blue mark. Bruises (without an underlying health cause) can happen by bumping into a door, a fall, or an accident such as my excited puppy lunging into my face.

What Scent-sational Oil Rx to Use: Make a topical mix of 3 drops of rosemary essential oil with 1 teaspoon of a carrier oil such as a light olive oil. Use twice a day until the bruises are gone.

Why You'll Essentially Feel Fine: The antioxidants in rosemary oil combined with anti-inflammatory lavender and chamomile oils can help relieve pain and swollen tissue. Also, olive oil as a carrier oil is a super antioxidant-rich oil with anti-inflammatory benefits. Using such a powerful essential oil blend with olive oil can help the bruise to fade and heal more quickly.

ESSENTIAL REMEDY #7: BURNS—HANDS ON THE BURN! THUMBS-UP TO CEDARWOOD.

A burn to your skin can happen anytime, anywhere. You can burn your hand on the stovetop or fireplace. And when you do, it hurts. First and foremost, after the burn happens you want to disinfect your skin to keep infection at bay.

What Scent-sational Oil Rx to Use: Try using a cedar citrus soap. Wash the burn with water and soap. Repeat as necessary.

Why You'll Essentially Feel Fine: There are a variety of cedar soaps available at online stores and aromatherapy shops. Some combine a variety of essential oils, including orange oil and rosemary oil. The healing components of cedar and orange oils include antioxidants, which act as an antiseptic to fight bacteria and can clean burns as well as abrasions, cuts, and sores to prevent infection. Not only is the soap easy to use, smells nice, it can help smooth and soothe the irritated and inflamed skin. One winter when I was stoking logs in the fireplace, a log dropped on my hand. My hand was red, blistered, and abraded. I ended up using peroxide to clean it, but if I could have a *Groundhog Day* re-do I'd use a cedar soap.

ESSENTIAL REMEDY #8: CANKER SORES—ZAP 'EM WITH LAVENDER!

Ouch! Symptoms of a small round sore inside the mouth can feel like a big pain! Canker sores occur for a variety of reasons, from emotional stress and acidic foods to an aggressive dental procedure. The upside is that while the inflammation can hurt, it will subside within ten days. Better yet, there is relief from an essential oil to help alleviate the hurt and speed up the recovery.

What Scent-sational Oil Rx to Use: If you apply 1 drop of lavender essential oil diluted with a dab of coconut oil to the affected area 2 times per day, it may reduce canker sore swelling and pain and even shorten the healing time.

Why You'll Essentially Feel Fine: Versatile lavender oil contains anti-bacterial and anti-inflammatory properties which can help aid in lessening an infection and pain. There are prescription dental pastes that do the same thing, but an essential oil remedy is cost-effective and readily available without a visit to the dentist.

ESSENTIAL REMEDY #9: COLDS—WHIFF LAVENDER TO STAY WELL!

During the fall and winter months when the temperature drops and we're indoors more and closer to people, colds are common. If your immune system has been compromised by not eating right, sleep deprivation, and stress, you could end up catching a cold if you're around someone who has been infected. But the right essential oil can help bolster your immunity.

What Scent-sational Oil Rx to Use: Try inhaling lavender oil in different ways. You can take a lavender-scented bath. Mix 3 drops of essential lavender oil with ¼ cup of jojoba or almond oil. Put the concoction into a tub filled with water.

Why You'll Essentially Feel Fine: Lavender is a calming bacteria-fighting essential oil. Its anti-inflammatory compounds can help to keep you safeguarded against microbes and fomites—the germs found on surfaces and the environment. Remember, lavender is one of the oils in the formula the thieves used to stay well during the bubonic plague. When we come into contact with these, we're more vulnerable to achoo! and may end up sick. By using lavender to boost our immune system, it can help keep us well.

ESSENTIAL REMEDY #10: COLD SORES—AVOID RED BUMPS! TRY LAVENDER.

Ever feel that tingle on your lip and soon see an unsightly red sore? Meet an unwelcome visitor called a cold sore. Simply put, it is an infection caused by the herpes virus. Stress or even the sun can trigger an outbreak.

What Scent-sational Oil Rx to Use: Try using 1 drop of lavender essential oil with 1 ounce olive oil. Put the mixture on a cotton ball and directly on the cold sore. Repeat two times per day.

Why You'll Essentially Feel Fine: Lavender boasts anti-inflammatory properties. One afternoon at a coffee shop in a store mall I joined my friend. I noticed the red, inflamed sore on her upper lip. When my eyes met hers, I sensed she was embarrassed as she covered the red bump with her hand. We ended up at The Body Shop where she purchased lavender essential oil premixed in a carrier oil that can be used to restore your skin. A few days later, the cold sore was history.

ESSENTIAL REMEDY #11: CONSTIPATION—AVOID IRREGULARITY! GO WITH CINNAMON.

Being irregular is uncomfortable and frustrating. Causes can vary, but changes such as colder weather, travel, medications, not eating enough fiber-rich foods or drinking too little water, and even stress can be culprits.

What Scent-sational Oil Rx to Use: Pour hot water into an 8- to 12-ounce mug. Add 1 drop of cinnamon essential oil. Repeat as needed.

Why You'll Essentially Feel Fine: Keeping hydrated is one way to stay regular. But sometimes we need extra help, and that's where cinnamon essential oil comes to the rescue. How does cinnamon work? Its compound linalool can relax the intestines and speed up a sluggish digestive system, much like a stimulant effect of coffee. This, in turn, can help you go and get your energy back on track.

ESSENTIAL REMEDY #12: COUGH—STOP THE TICKLE IN YOUR THROAT! SNIFF ROSEMARY.

When you have that irritating tickle in your throat and need to cough it's, well, irritating. A cough often occurs after a common cold, toxins in the environment, or other issues. If it's a minor cough, there is a natural essential oil remedy that may work for you.

What Scent-sational Oil Rx to Use: Combine 4 drops of rosemary essential oil into a diffuser or vaporizer. Or simply put the oil onto a handkerchief and take a whiff or two.

Why You'll Feel Essentially Fine: Rosemary can be an aid to lessen the need to cough with due credit to a compound called 1,8-cinole. It may be because the relaxant effect of rosemary calms the muscles in the respiratory system, preventing coughing. Also, this self-care treatment can be better than cough drops, which include sugar and other ingredients that you can't pronounce. Plus, if you have a vial of rosemary oil, it's just as quick to stop the hacking.

ESSENTIAL REMEDY #13: CUTS—DISINFECT THEM WITH TEA TREE!

A cut on your finger, arm, or leg is not uncommon and can happen to anyone at any time. If the cut isn't deep and stops bleeding, chances are you will not require stitches. But that doesn't make the throbbing stop, and the healing process surely won't happen in minutes. There is an essential oil remedy that can help speed up the recovery process.

What Scent-sational Oil Rx to Use: Opt for tea tree oil diluted with apple cider vinegar. Use 3 to 5 drops of tea tree oil mixed with ¼ cup vinegar. Use a cotton ball and dab the wound. Repeat three times per day.

Why You'll Essentially Feel Fine: Folk remedy experts explain that 5 percent solution of tea tree oil can work as good as a 5 percent benzoyl peroxide medication. Also, there may be less burning and redness during the healing process.[1]

Adds the co-founder of Kobashi Essential Oil Company, Lynda Ballard, "Tea tree is a great antiseptic. We always have it on hand to treat cuts. It also works great with lavender. In fact, we blend the two oils into aloe vera in our first-aid roller balls."

ESSENTIAL REMEDY #14: DIZZINESS—STAY GROUNDED WITH CHAMOMILE!

Eek! When you're light-headed sometimes the world can feel like it's spinning out of control. Dizziness can happen without warning, and it can be caused by a number of reasons, including anxiety, dehydration, prescription drugs, or abrupt withdrawal from some medications. Knowing the reason is helpful because it can help you to cope and find a way to get grounded. Once you discover the culprit behind your dizziness, you can address the cause accordingly.,

What Scent-sational Oil Rx to Use: Put 1 drop of chamomile essential oil diluted with 1 teaspoon honey in a 12-ounce cup of hot water and drink it. Plus, wearing an aromatic jewelry necklace with a few drops of sandalwood on a pad can be an extra gesture to help you feel on even keel, whether you're on a boat, plane, or at home and feeling light-headed.

Why You'll Essentially Feel Fine: Chamomile and its calming compounds are known to help calm and stave off or treat anxiety. Anxiety often comes with a feeling of light-headedness, which can make you feel unsteady. Also, dehydration can leave you feeling dizzy as well.

ESSENTIAL REMEDY #15: DRY SKIN—SMOOTH LIZARD SKIN! CHAMOMILE IT UP!

Dry skin is not life-threatening, but it can be bothersome and even painful. There are natural essential oils that can help to heal the effects of weathered skin, such as dry hands and cuticles, a constant challenge I cope with during cold winters.

What Scent-sational Oil Rx to Use: Combine 3 drops chamomile essential oil and 2 drops sandalwood oil in ¼ ounce all-natural unscented lotion or olive oil. Rub the lotion directly on affected areas. Repeat twice each day.

Why You'll Essentially Feel Fine: Southern California–based luxury Cal-a-Vie spa director says that chamomile essential oil can be beneficial to treat an array of skin conditions, which include cracked dry skin, inflamed skin, and eczema. Chamomile contains anti-inflammatory properties that help remedy the effects of dry skin and make it feel softer and smoother, healing crevices and cracks.

Naturopath & Aromatherapist Sascha Beck explains that sandalwood oil can be helpful for dry skin because of its anti-inflammatory and moisturizing properties. "My favorite use is to blend it with other essential oils in a face potion," she says.

A Bonus: Dry cuticles are a challenge I battle every winter. Especially due to the dry, cold climate, chemicals at the resort swimming pool and hot tub, shoveling snow, and making fires. Tea tree oil mixed with an all-natural unscented lotion keeps bacterial infections away and quickly heals the cracked skin around my fingers. I use 2 drops of tea tree oil with ¼ ounce of lotion or jojoba oil.

ESSENTIAL REMEDY #16: EARACHE—SOOTHE THE THROBBING WITH LAVENDER AND OLIVE OIL!

A mild earache can be an annoyance. Often, it can be due to swimmer's ear. If this is the case, it can be tended to with self-care at home. And that's when the essential oil lavender comes to your aid.

What Scent-sational Oil Rx to Use: Try mixing 1 drop of lavender essential oil with 2 drops of olive oil. Use a cotton ball and apply the oil solution around the ear canal. Repeat 2 to 3 times daily.

Why You'll Essentially Feel Fine: Lavender oil contains anti-inflammatory and antibacterial properties. This, in result, may calm an earache due to bacteria such as in swimmer's ear. Olive oil, much like lavender oil, also contains anti-inflammatory and antibacterial properties. In fact, you may not need prescription ear drops and your ears can heal, naturally.

ESSENTIAL REMEDY #17: FATIGUE—GET ENERGIZED! INHALE LEMON AND ROSEMARY.

There can be many causes for tiredness, including sleep deprivation, traveling, or working day and night without breaks. Essential oils won't be as healthful as a good night's sleep or a much needed vacation, but the right oils can give you a temporary lift.

What Scent-sational Oil to Use: In a plastic container, combine 1 drop lemon oil and 1 drop rosemary oil in an all-natural bath soap or unscented gel. Take a hot shower.

Why You'll Essentially Feel Fine: You will feel invigorated by these two essential oils. Refreshing citrus oil's antioxidants help invigorate mood and uplift your spirit, whereas stacks of past research show rosemary oil can enhance mental alertness and mood. The steam from the shower will aid in circulating the vapor, too. Aromatic stimulants can boost our mood and spirit, as well as the relaxing hydrotherapy. Unlike sugary soft drinks or caffeinated energy drinks, these natural oils will help you feel rejuvenated and maintain that sense of balance without a crash like sugar or caffeine.

ESSENTIAL REMEDY #18: FEVER—COOL DOWN! COMPRESS WITH CHAMOMILE.

A low-grade fever is not uncommon if you're coming down with a cold or flu. If your temperature rises a bit (not more than 101) it could be a wait-and-see situation rather than an E.R. moment. A fever is often our body's way of trying to fight off an infection.

What Scent-sational Oil to Use: Mix 3 to 4 drops of chamomile oil to 1 pint of water. Use a washcloth and give yourself a soothing sponge bath, including your face, chest, arms, and legs. Drink plenty of water and herbal tea as well as rest.

Why You'll Essentially Feel Fine: Your temperature may likely go down to normal within 24 hours. Chamomile essential oil is nature's anti-inflammatory, much like ibuprofen we take for aches and pains. One late spring I ended up with a mild sinus infection. When the thermometer hit 100, I made a doctor's appointment. She ended up giving me a prescription for antibiotics but also said that my situation would have gone away by itself and self-care.

ESSENTIAL REMEDY #19: FIBROMYALGIA—SOOTHE ACHES WITH EUCALYPTUS!

Aches and pains in your muscles can be due to fibromyalgia or fibrositis. There are eighteen tender points that will determine if you do have fibromyalgia; however, not all people will have issues with each one. If you have mild achy muscles after over exertion, during cold weather, or a bout of stress, it can cause a fibromyalgia flare-up. Taking an essential oil route may work wonders.

What Scent-sational Oil Rx to Use: Combine ¼ cup of unscented, natural lotion. Add 2 drops of eucalyptus oil and mix well. Rub the cream into your skin. Repeat as needed.

Why You'll Essentially Feel Fine: In the wintertime after shoveling snow, bringing in firewood, and walking the dog in snow, taking a hot shower loosens up tight muscles. Massaging your muscles with a eucalyptus oil–based lotion with its eucalyptol compound will tingle and numb painful muscle tissue, and create blood circulation.

ESSENTIAL REMEDY #20: GUM ISSUES—KEEP GUMS HEALTHY! KISS PEPPERMINT HELLO.

Gingivitis is a gum disease that causes inflamed and swollen gums. Sometimes they can ache or even bleed when brushing and flossing. If you're neglecting regular brushing and flossing, this can be a cause. Hormones and/or stress can affect your gums, too. But don't despair. There is help, naturally, with an essential oil.

What Scent-sational Oil Rx to Use: Put 2 drops of peppermint essential oil into an 8-ounce glass of warm water. Rinse with the solution. Follow with a thorough tooth brushing.

Why You'll Essentially Feel Fine: Peppermint oil is often an ingredient found in different toothpastes. Past research and anecdotal evidence has shown that essential oils, including peppermint oil, may help fight bacteria and germs, thanks to their antimicrobial action that provides an antiseptic (like a store-bought or prescription mouthwash) to fight bacteria.

ESSENTIAL REMEDY #21: HEADACHES—WRAP UP THE ACHE, A CHAMOMILE FIX!

Ugh. A throbbing headache has paid you a visit. It can be a tension headache, which aches in the forehead area; sinus headaches can be felt between the eyes and/or forehead; and abrupt caffeine withdrawal can make your entire head ache! Whatever the cause, a headache can be painful and distracting, which is why you'll need chamomile oil to get you back on track!

What Scent-sational Oil Rx to Use: Mix 5 drops of chamomile essential oil and $\frac{1}{2}$ cup cold water into a small bowl. Use a washcloth as an icepack-type compress. Soak it into the oil and water solution and place on your forehead for about 5 minutes. Repeat as necessary.

Why You'll Essentially Feel Fine: The aching of a nagging tension headache, the most common type, will subside. Give credit to the chamomile oil, which is an anti-inflammatory like ibuprofen. Combined with cold water it can help to alleviate inflamed blood vessels and offer you a quick remedy to being headache-free.

ESSENTIAL REMEDY #22: HEARTBURN—SOOTHE YOUR GI TRACT THE CHAMOMILE WAY!

Oh, the scourge of heartburn can be worse than heartache . . . or so it seems. If you get occasional heartburn it is most likely due to the foods you ate. Rich, fatty foods like poultry with a sauce, acidic tomato sauce, onions, and garlic are triggers for me, as is overindulging in food or alcohol. Heartburn can be caused by a spasm in the stomach or it can occur when the esophagus creates acid from your stomach that moves up the throat. Usually, it will go away overnight, but it is uncomfortable and you'll find yourself reaching for an antacid. But what if you don't have any in the house?

What Scent-sational Oil to Use: Make a massage oil. Mix 3 drops of chamomile essential oil and 1 ounce of olive oil. Rub on your heart and clavicle. Also, drinking a cup of hot chamomile tea flavored with 1 drop of lemon oil can soothe your pain.

Why You'll Essentially Feel Fine: Lemons contain citric acid and ascorbic acid, two compounds that can help soothe heartburn and indigestion. One autumn, I was craving hot salsa with tortilla chips. Instead of making the sauce (mistake one), I purchased a store-bought brand with garlic (mistake two) since the regular type was sold out. It was flavorful but I ended up eating too much (mistake three). At 1:00 A.M., when the ruthless heartburn monster woke me up, the chamomile remedy with citrus oil really worked. I fell back to sleep.

ESSENTIAL REMEDY #23: HEMORRHOIDS—SOOTHE YOUR BUM! CHAMOMILE HEALS.

Internal or external hemorrhoids can affect almost everyone sooner or later. The blood vessels in the lower part of your bottom can become inflamed and irritated. Pregnancy, straining during a bowel movement, and sitting for long periods of time can all be causes of this usually temporary pain in the bottom.

What Scent-sational Oil to Use: Dilute equal parts of chamomile essential oil with an oil such as jojoba oil. Use a clean compress and place on the bottom. Repeat two or three times per day.

Why You'll Essentially Feel Fine: The soothing effects of anti-inflammatory chamomile oil can help shrink the swelling of the irritated blood vessels. One time I was prescribed antibiotics after a root canal. After two cycles of the medication, I began to suffer from diarrhea. Then, mild bleeding followed and gave me a scare. But my doctor assured me it was a side effect of the medication. My friend brought me a care package of over-the-counter hemorrhoid creams and pads. In hindsight, I wish I had known that a simple, soothing folk remedy like calming chamomile and water could have been the answer to soothe my ailing rear end.

ESSENTIAL REMEDY #24: HYPOCHONDRIA—NIX NEGATIVE THOUGHTS. SMELL THE ROSES!

Hypochondria is a mental disorder in which you imagine you may have a health ailment or serious disease, causing major anxiety. Medical students and even health authors, like me, can study the symptoms of various health issues and soon begin to believe we have it—whatever it is.

What Scent-sational Oil Rx to Use: Combine 3 drops of rose oil into a diffuser filled with water. Inhale the oil and water air for about 15 to 30 minutes. You can also use lavender or chamomile because these oils are less pricey.

Why You'll Essentially Feel Fine: Both essential oils, lavender and rose, are calming due to their fragrant floral scent. Also, these scents can boost blood circulation, which is useful for lower blood pressure. The Fourth of July is a particularly intense and loud holiday and on top of all that, one year, I agonized when standing in line at the grocery store behind a tourist who was coughing and sneezing. The next day I pondered, "I think I'm coming down with a cold." I was imitating Harry Burns's character in the classic romantic comedy *When Harry Met Sally*. I put rose oil and water in the diffuser and turned up the white noise—fans, stereo, and air purifier. The end result: I was relaxed during the bangs and booms of the fireworks and concerts. My energy helped keep the dog and cat on an even keel. We survived.

ESSENTIAL REMEDY #25: INATTENTIVE—GET FOCUSED! IT'S LEMON TIME.

Feeling distracted can affect your mood. If you're having problems paying attention it might be caused by anxiety and stress. Scent, however, can turn mental blocks around and help to boost mood, attention span, and alertness.

What Scent-sational Oil Rx to Use: Try an aromatic pottery diffuser. It's portable and easy to use at home in different rooms. Fill the diffuser with 5 drops of lemon essential oil. Or try a vaporizer filled with water (follow the directions for how much) and add 2 drops of lemon oil and breathe in the oil.

Why You'll Essentially Feel Fine: Past research in the Japanese workplace used citrusy lemon fragrance in the morning hours to help stimulate the minds of workers. Lemon oil can uplift your spirits. Inhaling the citrus scent triggers norepinephrine and that increases heart rate, as well as boosts mental and physical activity so you are more apt to be attentive.

ESSENTIAL REMEDY #26: INSECT BITES—TAKE THE STING AWAY! SPRITZ PEPPERMINT.

Bees, spiders, wasps—oh my! When a bug bites your skin, it can smart and burn. Identifying the insect is important for safety's sake because sometimes a tetanus shot may be necessary. Then, it's time to deal with the redness and swelling.

What Scent-sational Oil Rx to Use: In a small spray bottle, combine 2 drops of peppermint essential oil with 1 ounce of witch hazel. Witch hazel should be available at your drugstore or health food store and it's best to have in your medicine cabinet. Spritz the bite(s) with the solution.

Why You'll Essentially Feel Fine: Peppermint oil contains anti-inflammatory and antibacterial properties. The menthol ingredient in it will create a tingling effect, which may feel like it's counteracting the pain, sort of like a numbing cream the dental hygienist may use on your gum to lessen the pain of a dental cleaning. In my hiking days, during my twenties, I recall getting stranded on a road in Florida in a region called Alligator Alley. It was hot and humid. As I was obsessed with alligators and snakes—that wasn't the challenge. I felt like a victim in a spooky sci-fi film Attack of the Killer Mosquitoes! I was rescued by a truck driver from the South. She took out her first-aid kit and handed me a vial of peppermint oil for my bites. I applied the potion with cotton balls. I was amazed and thankful for the Southern hospitality and the healing powers of the minty oil.

Lavender, ANOTHER BUGS-OFF PLUS Essential Oil

Naturopath & Aromatherapist Sascha Beck, of Perth, Western Australia, shares in her own words her appreciation for lavender oil, not peppermint, her choice of essential oil to survive an adventure or misadventure . . .

If I could only take one essential oil to a desert island, natural disaster, glamping, traveling, or just going on a walk-about, it would be lavender—*Lavandula angustifolia* to be precise! It is the best remedy I have ever found for taking the sting and itch out of mosquito bites. Try a dilution of 0.5 ounces (15 mL) of lavender oil with 3 ounces (85 mL) of aloe vera gel on insect bites, small scratches, grazes, and minor burns. For sunburn, which covers larger areas of the body, try 1 teaspoon (5 mL) of lavender oil with 3 ounces (85 mL) aloe vera gel.

Lavender repels many creepy-crawlies and has significant antimicrobial activity. Diluted with a base oil its anti-inflammatory and analgesic effects are helpful for relieving achy muscles and joints, relaxing the nervous system, helping to reduce anxiety, and assisting with sleep. It is a first-aid kit in a sweet-smelling bottle!

Note: If you are using lavender oil for its medicinal properties, there are a number of different species used in aromatherapy oils and each species has a different chemical composition—and therefore slightly different therapeutic indications.

ESSENTIAL REMEDY #27: INSOMNIA—CUDDLE UP TO A GERANIUM MASSAGE!

Not getting enough shut-eye is a major problem for people, according to the National Sleep Foundation. We need adequate sleep to help restore our body and mind. Lack of sleep causes stress, poor eating habits, and wears down our immune system.

What Scent-sational Oil Rx to Use: Try a solo self-massage with a geranium essential oil blend. Mix 2 drops of geranium with 1 drop each of chamomile and lavender in about 4 ounces of an all-natural unscented lotion. Rub gently on your neck, arms, belly, and legs.

Why You'll Essentially Feel Fine: Geranium, like lavender essential oil, is popular for its calming and mood-stabilizing properties, including its linalool compound. Dr. Ann Louise Gittleman's go-to oil is lavender to get some sleep. I personally prefer swimming during the day, a cup of chamomile tea at night, and this geranium massage lotion as a perfect nightcap.

ESSENTIAL REMEDY #28: IRRITABLE BOWEL SYNDROME— TRICK YOUR TUMMY! PEPPERMINT CURES.

People who have experienced irritable bowel syndrome or IBS know all too well that coping with irregularity can be uncomfortable. I will never forget during my under-graduate school days when I got up close and personal with my earthy nutrition teacher who lived in a commune with other teachers. After class I told her the news.

"I think I ate too much fiber foods. I'm still irregular and bloated. It's not working."

She asked, "Are you drinking water?"

I shook my head and said, "I forgot."

She advised staying hydrated and try the all-natural peppermint oil cure.

What Scent-sational Oil Rx to Use: Put 1 drop of essential peppermint oil into a cup of hot water once per day as needed.

Why You'll Essentially Feel Fine: Peppermint oil can help with tummy troubles if consumed with water. The main component is menthol, which may relax the smooth muscle in the small intestine and lessen stomach cramps and spasms.[2]

ESSENTIAL REMEDY #29: JET LAG—FEEL NORMAL—AND ENERGIZED. ORANGE UP!

Traveling far or even not so far but out of your time zone can wear on your body and mind. It's an irritating feeling of sleeplessness and fatigue, sort of like staying up all night long. It's tempting to crave a caffeine drink to feel normal, but then you won't get back into the rhythm the next day. A natural remedy is turning to an essential oil to feel more alert, more energized so you can go with the flow until your circadian clock adjusts, much like when we turn the clocks forward or backward during spring and fall.

What Scent-sational Oil Rx to Use: Make a mixture of 1 drop of orange essential oil with 1 teaspoon carrier oil like almond or jojoba. Put a dab on your wrist or clavicle.

Why You'll Essentially Feel Fine: Citrus oil has been proven to trigger chemicals that can trick your brain into an energized state. Not only will you feel more alert and in a better mood, this natural remedy just may be the answer to avoiding caffeine and fighting the lag until you are back and enjoying the trip. Ann, a friend of mine who lives in Norway, turns to nature's oil(s) during seasonal change. "I use the citrus and cinnamon as a pick-me-up," she says, "when there are just four hours of daylight during the winter it can feel like constant jet lag." The natural oils can help you to feel more normal until your body adjusts to the change of hours, light and dark.

ESSENTIAL REMEDY #30: LOW LIBIDO—SMELL THAT LOVING FEELING WITH SANDALWOOD, SWEETIE!

Both women and men can experience a lack of sex drive during different times in their lives. It can be due to depression, hormones, stress, and even aging. Often these factors are temporary and libido returns, naturally—or even with a little bit of help from essential oils.

What Scent-sational Oil Rx to Use: Put 1 drop of sandalwood essential oil mixed with 1 drop of jojoba oil directly on your wrist or take a whiff of the oil from a vial.

Why You'll Essentially Feel Fine: Kurt Schnaubelt of Pacific Institute of Aromatherapy, in San Rafael, California, touts the earthy scent for its ability to "improve mood" perhaps due to its "warm and uplifting" therapeutic nature. Its fragrance is believed to boost self-confidence, which is a turn-on for men and women. In my forties, I experienced the dating scene after the end of a long relationship. I remember wearing sandalwood oil that I purchased from The Body Shop. A dab of sandalwood on my wrist made me feel like an approachable natural woman, like wearing mascara or lip gloss. I felt stark-naked without wearing it. The essential oil made me feel complete, and sandalwood was my signature scent.

Scent of a Wo(man)

Aromatherapists believe some essential oils can incite sexual desire. History shows scent and sex are often coupled so to speak. According to sex therapists and medical doctors, sex is healthy. Sex triggers physiological changes to the nervous system, much like exercise. Feel-good endorphins are released and we can feel calmer. So, what essential oils can help boost your sex drive and help you to feel in the mood to make love?

The top romantic oils include jasmine, rose, and sandalwood. These three essential oils have a history of being touted as sensual oils for people in the past. Wearing oils like rose absolute can make you feel oh-so sensual, like booking a room at a five-star hotel. But inexpensive oils like patchouli and sandalwood can help you lose inhibitions, allowing you to feel centered and confident. Not to forget, having cinnamon rolls baking in the oven or vanilla-scented candles lit can set the mood for a couple as it often triggers feel-good memories and nostalgia.

ESSENTIAL REMEDY #31: MENOPAUSAL HOT FLASHES—COOL DOWN! SPRITZ YOURSELF WITH PEPPERMINT.

If you have a hot flash you will know it. For years during "The Change" I didn't experience one. Until one sobering day. At a book signing I, the ambivert author, was sipping a cup of hot tea and talking to customers. *Bam!* I felt my face heat up and was told it was red, like a blushing teenager. It was my first hot flash. It subsided on its own. If I could go back in time an essential oil could have helped me to chill.

What Scent-sational Oil Rx to Use: In a small spritzer bottle combine 5 drops of peppermint essential oil with one ounce of water. Or combine 1 drop of jojoba oil and 1 drop of peppermint oil. Once a sudden hot flash hits, simply spritz your face with the liquid potion.

Why You'll Essentially Feel Fine: Hot flashes are due to a fluctuation in hormones, and stress or heat can be triggers. How does peppermint work to quell the uncomfortable feeling? Medical research shows peppermint oil may help boost up calmness. One middle-aged woman I know copes with hot flashes by using peppermint oil. She puts one drop of peppermint oil (she only uses the doTerra brand) under her tongue or mists her face with a solution of peppermint oil and water. She insists it provides instant relief.

ESSENTIAL REMEDY #32: MIGRAINE—STOP THE THROBBING! COOL IT WITH PEPPERMINT.

Headaches are uncomfortable, but a migraine is the grandmother of headaches. Not only can it cause excruciating pain on one side of your head, but light sensitivity and nausea can make getting a migraine miserable. Most likely, you will be willing to try a self-care remedy to drive the ill effects away.

What Scent-sational Oil Rx to Use: Try mixing 5 drops of peppermint oil in a quart of hot water. Place a clean washcloth into the solution and use it as a compress for 15 minutes. Repeat as needed.

Why You'll Essentially Feel Fine: Thanks to the menthol compound in peppermint oil, it can help relax muscles and alleviate pain. A study published in *Frontiers in Neurology* showed that the minty oil with healing powers can stop a migraine by using a topical gel with six percent of menthol. More research is necessary but if an occasional migraine pays you an untimely visit you may want to give it a try.[3]

ESSENTIAL REMEDY #33: PANIC ATTACK—CHILL! USE A CHAMOMILE COMPRESS.

Panic attacks can happen without warning. There are a variety of reasons as to why the attacks can occur. It can happen due to hormones gone haywire (such as during peri-menopause), drug withdrawal, or stressful life events. The nervous system is out of whack and your heart rate increases. You can get irrational thoughts, even possibly believing you're having a heart attack. The bottom line: If you have a panic attack it is usually not life-threatening but extremely unsettling. If you feel high stress or anxiety, it may be time to take action and you may be able to prevent it.

What Scent-sational Oil Rx to Use: Wear an aromatic jewelry necklace. Always have a calming essential oil on the pad inside it. Chamomile is an excellent choice, as is sandalwood and lavender. Or put a cold compress on your forehead soaked in 4 drops of chamomile and 4 drops of jojoba oil.

Why You'll Essentially Feel Fine: If you take a whiff or two or three of calming chamomile oil when you start feeling anxious, it may nip a potential panic attack from happening. Pairing this remedy with other essential oils may help, too. Sandalwood boosts confidence and lavender induces a sense of calm. Once you've inhaled, try to distract yourself in order to lure your brain away from your panicked thinking. In a Hallmark film one character was stressed out by trying to do too much for a holiday event. A doctor's keen observation of the oncoming panic attack was diverted by him asking her to recite the song, "The Twelve

Days of Christmas." So, forget the paper bag trick. Instead, inhale chamomile, take deep breaths, and distract, distract, distract.

ESSENTIAL REMEDY #34: PMS CRAMPS—RUB AWAY ACHES THE PEPPERMINT WAY!

Pre-menstrual cramps and crankies are "the curse" for women in their child-bearing years. While both go hand in hand, there is help for cramps that I didn't know about during those days and nights when I used a heating pad and the mantra, "Go away."

What Scent-sational Rx Oil to Use: Try using a self-massage on top of the pelvic region. Combine ¼ cup of carrier oil such as jojoba oil or almond oil with 2 drops of peppermint essential oil. Also, while relaxing, sip 1 cup of hot water with 1 drop of chamomile essential oil.

Why You'll Essentially Feel Fine: Aromatherapists will tell you peppermint oil contains both anti-inflammatory and antispasmodic properties. These compounds can likely help relax the pelvic pain. Chamomile essential oil with its calming benefits will also calm your irritable mood.

ESSENTIAL REMEDY #35: POISON OAK/IVY—TAME THE ITCH! WHIP IT WITH LAVENDER.

If you get too close to poison oak or ivy plants in the great outdoors, you may end up with an unwanted condition soon after. Itching, redness, swelling, and blisters are the name of the poison plant game, and it's one that isn't fun to play. As a kid I developed a terrible case, which almost landed me in the hospital. When I was in my late teens, I fell victim once again to the plant and paid the price. Worse, I didn't try the essential oil remedy.

What Scent-sational Oil to Use: In a small container, combine 4 drops of lavender oil and 1 tablespoon of apple cider vinegar. Dip a washcloth into the mixture and dab the compress on affected skin. Repeat as necessary.

Why You'll Essentially Feel Fine: The wonder of this home cure is that the oil and vinegar do not shroud the unsightly sores on your skin. I used pink calamine lotion in my youth, and it made me look like a monster from a pastel planet. If I had known about lavender oil and vinegar, I wouldn't have appeared hideous and its healing properties could have worked just as well. Lavender's anti-inflammatory benefits in combination with vinegar's acetic acid (the compound that clears up warts and blemishes) can fight swelling, redness, infection, and dry up sores.

ESSENTIAL REMEDY #36: SEASONAL AFFECTIVE DISORDER— PEP UP! FEEL HAPPIER WITH VANILLA.

When Old Man Winter arrives with shorter days and longer nights, the darkness may affect you—and a low mood may be an unwanted visitor. Seasonal Affective Disorder (SAD) affects millions of people, but nature's sweetest aromatic essential oil can be beneficial.

What Scent-sational Oil Rx to Use: Bundle up and burn an all-natural vanilla candle or incense stick in the bathroom. Mix 5 drops of vanilla essential oil with 5 drops of jojoba or almond oil. Put into a full bathtub of water and soak.

Why You'll Essentially Feel Fine: Historians tell us that in the fifteenth century people used vanilla to cope with low mood, which can come with stress and worry. The main compound in vanilla essential oil is vanillin; it can rev up feel-good hormones naturally and may help you feel more like you and bounce back.

ESSENTIAL REMEDY #37: SINUSITUS—CLEAR YOUR HEAD! BREATHE EUCALYPTUS.

A bout of sinusitis comes with a mixed bag of symptoms. Congestion and a headache are common. It can happen during seasonal changes, such as the fall and spring when the pollen count is high. Sinus problems also can occur in a dry climate.

What Scent-sational Oil Rx to Use: For a quick stovetop steam put 3 drops of eucalyptus oil in 2 cups of water in a pan; simmer the liquid until it is hot. Turn off the heat. Place your face over the steam and use a towel over your head. Repeat as needed.

Why You'll Essentially Feel Fine: I've been a survivor of sinusitis for years. The symptoms are often a sinus headache and congestion. One January day I revisited my dentist for pain near the back upper right molar.

"Is the tooth cracked?" I asked.

"No," answered the doctor.

"Do I have an abscess?"

"No," he said.

He told me the pain could be due to my sinuses. A few days later, after trying the eucalyptus remedy in a diffuser, the ache was gone. I give credit to the oil's compound eucalyptol. Aromatherapists know that eucalyptus can help clear sinuses by lessening both inflammation and congestion. This home cure is fairly quick and provides fast results.

Sniff Sinus Woes Away!

If you're still suffering from painful sinuses, try this essential oil blend. The combination of the oils may just be nature's perfect prescription for you.

4 drops lemon essential oil
4 drops peppermint essential oil
4 drops lavender essential oil
4 drops eucalyptus essential oil
1 to 2 ounces of carrier oil

Try this blend in a roller ball, or in a room diffuser or bath. For bath and skin applications, dilute mixture with 1 to 2 ounces of carrier oil such as grape seed, sweet almond, or jojoba oils.

(Courtesy: LorAnn Oils)

ESSENTIAL REMEDY #38: SORE THROAT—LOSE SCRATCHINESS ASAP! LEMON, BABY.

Ouch! A sore throat is an unwelcome irritation of scratchy pain when you talk and swallow. It can be a sign that you may be coming down with a cold or flu. Or it could be caused by allergies, strep throat, or even talking too much—which can result in laryngitis or even polyps on the larynx!

What Scent-sational Oil Rx to Use: Try putting 1 drop of lemon oil in 8 ounces of hot water. Add 1 teaspoon raw honey for taste. Repeat twice daily.

Why You'll Essentially Feel Fine: Lemon oil is known for its action to rid the body of toxins, due to its antioxidant vitamin C. The oil has antibacterial and anti-inflammatory properties. This popular essential oil also may trigger saliva, which can help keep the throat hydrated. In my thirties, I ended up seeing an ear, nose, and throat specialist. The diagnosis? I had developed calluses on my larynx, and was told it was from excessive talking. I used the lemon oil, honey, and water remedy. I was back to chatting within a few days.

ESSENTIAL REMEDY #39: SPRAINS—RUB A SORE LIMB. PRACTICE EUCALYPTUS MAGIC!

An injury to the body's ligaments that connect your muscles to your bones is a sprain. There are different levels of a sprain, but if it is sore, and mild bruising occurs after, usually time will heal it. Self-care with essential oil can help speed up the recovery time.

What Scent-sational Oil Rx to Use: Add 4 drops of eucalyptus essential oil to ¼ ounce jojoba oil. Massage the sprained area 2 to 3 times daily.

Why You'll Essentially Feel Fine: Eucalyptus oil can numb the pain of a mild sprain. Its anti-inflammatory properties penetrate into the ligaments and your sore muscles. Case-in-point: One early afternoon, after walking the dog, answering the phone, and getting ready to swim, I was simply distracted. In the living room as I headed toward the front door, I tripped but caught myself on the love seat and broke the fall. But my left ankle still twisted. By nighttime, my ankle was swollen and throbbed. And that's when I turned to the eucalyptus method, which soothed the aching and swelling. In days I was healed.

ESSENTIAL REMEDY #40: STRESS—RESTORE THE CALM! COZY UP TO LAVENDER.

Welcome to stress, which can be the scourge for people of all ages. Turning to fragrant essential oils can help lighten up your pressures. Specific essential oils can help alleviate stress-related symptoms, including anxiety and even tension headaches.

What Scent-sational Oil Rx to Use: In a small glass vial, combine 1 ounce of almond oil with 1 drop each of lavender and vanilla essential oils. Massage into skin, including arms, legs, and back. Lighting a scented candle of one of these scents can be helpful, too.

Why You'll Essentially Feel Fine: Stress overload can zap energy, "cause wear and tear on the body," leaving you prone to "illness and premature aging," points out Reneau Z. Peurifoy, M.A., author of *Anxiety, Phobias, & Panic*. He notes, massage can be beneficial for people suffering from stress because it can help ease muscle tension and it's a good form of relaxation.[4]

Using a destressing vanilla oil formula, you get a massage using essential oils to stimulate the lymphatic system and calm the nervous system. Spa therapists believe lavender essential oil used in a massage can help guests to unwind and relax when used on the skin.

Rub-On Essential Oils for Shingles Support

I've known people, mostly elderly friends, who have endured an outbreak of shingles, a skin condition that often strikes on the back or face, especially during or after coping with a stressful event. It is believed that if you've had chicken pox before and your immune system is down, you are more likely to experience a shingles occurrence.

Lynda Ballard of Kobashi Essential Oils tells her tale of shingles.

When my father died suddenly, I came down with a case of shingles. I quickly put together a mix of geranium, lavender, oregano, tea tree, sandalwood, and thyme, in a blend of carrier oils of grape seed, infused calendula, and St. John's Wort, which we grow organically.

I massaged this blend morning and night and thankfully the shingles only lasted a few weeks and never spread or re-appeared.

ESSENTIAL REMEDY #41: TONGUE BURN—PAMPER IT! TRY LAVENDER OIL, BABY.

Imagine this scenario. You mindlessly wolf down a slice of hot pizza or sip a cup of hot tea. Ouch! You burned the tip of your tongue. The upside? It will heal within a few days or up to one week—and faster if you take the essential oil route.

What Scent-sational Oil Rx to Use: Mix 1 drop of lavender oil with 1 drop of light olive oil. Repeat twice daily.

Why You'll Essentially Feel Fine: Lavender oil contains anti-inflammatory compounds and so does olive oil. The combination should lessen the redness and burning you feel on the tender tongue. It is best to stay clear of acidic and crunchy foods until your tongue burn heals—and it will. One night I was multitasking. The telephone rang. I grabbed a dish of spinach cheese ravioli and ate it mindlessly while talking on the phone—and ignoring the steam rising from the pasta. Soon after, I realized that I burned the tip of my tongue. That night I turned to soothing lavender essential oil and olive oil and found it to be quite an easy natural remedy.

ESSENTIAL REMEDY #42: TOOTHACHE—AVOID UNBEARABLE PAIN WITH CLOVE!

Clove oil is nothing new as a remedy to quell an aching tooth. A toothache can be caused by an abscess, a gum infection, a cavity, grinding your teeth, or even sinuses. Whatever the culprit, when a tooth throbs, a temporary home cure is more than welcome—until you can make it to the dentist.

What Scent-sational Oil Rx to Use: Mix 1 drop of clove essential oil with 3 drops of light olive oil. Apply the oil mixture directly on the tooth. Repeat as necessary.

Why You'll Essentially Feel Fine: One night I was munching on a dried fig. When I bit down on the dried fruit, I heard a loud crunch. A tiny piece of my last upper molar had chipped off. The pain was intense. Since I couldn't get an appointment until the next morning, I resorted to the chilling *Marathon Man* film's "clove of oils" for numbing the pain as used by actor Dustin Hoffman whose character had his tooth drilled into the dentin without the use of Novocain.

Clove oil contains eugenol, touted for its antiseptic and pain-relieving properties that can numb gums. This method was used in the past.

ESSENTIAL REMEDY #43: UNIVERSAL E.R. CONDITIONS— STOCK UP! GET YOUR OILS IN A ROW.

The thing is, we never know when a natural or man-made disaster can strike. Often, an earthquake, wildfire, and power outage happen without much foreshadow. Most of us have survived an emergency, but not all of us have a good emergency stockpile, especially with essential oils. To make it easy, I am selecting one oil that seems to be one of the most popular and versatile to own.

What Scent-sational Oil Rx to Use: Store a vial of lavender oil and a bottle of olive oil, my carrier oil of choice.

Why You'll Essentially Feel Fine: Lavender oil contains linalool, which can relax you. Plus, its anti-inflammatory and antibacterial compounds have you covered for anxiety, cuts, stomach disorders, stress, wounds, and more drama disorders. During the San Francisco Earthquake on October 17, 1989, I experienced a 7.1 major quake. I ran for the doorway but fell because the floor was buckling in waves, making it impossible to stand. I cut my leg and feet. No first-aid kit. These days, lavender essential oil is my first-aid essential oil when disaster strikes.

Healing Oils—Essential First-Aid Kit

During a disaster, a first-aid kit is a must-have. Having a ready-to-use supply of essential oils could be a welcoming surprise for you and yours. There are more than three hundred healing oils. The Pacific Institute of Aromatherapy's founder, Kurt Schnaubelt, chose a variety of oils that could be put into your first-aid kit. He states, "There are six essential oils that have a good amount of human usage, which attests to their usefulness and safety." Drum roll. His picks include lavender, lemon, melissa, peppermint, rosemary, and thyme—four in my top 20 essential oils.

I asked Dr. Ann Louise Gittleman the question:

"If you were stranded on a desert island, what one essential oil would you want to have with you?"

She answered, myrrh would be her "go-to for body, mind, spirit healing, and soothing soft tissue injuries." The doctor added, jojoba would be her carrier oil of choice.

I put together this list of essential oils for a disaster kit, for me, and perhaps you, too. Back to the scenario where we are on our own, whether it is a *Survivor Island*–type of challenge or a disaster has struck. Here are my recommendations for your go-to essential oils first-aid kit:

✓ Lavender: This oil, as noted before, is number one in my book to calm anxiety and stress during day-to-day life's ups and downs to a real disaster. It can be inhaled and used topically.

✓ Lemon: A citrusy oil to help keep you alert and uplift your spirits if feeling fatigued or depressed. This essential oil can be inhaled from the vial.

✓ Peppermint: During tough times, digestion woes can hit. This minty oil can help soothe your stomach if you're nervous, or calm your tummy if you have to eat ants or frogs or worse!

✓ Rosemary: A wonderful anti-inflammatory and antibacterial oil, this is ideal for skin care, from burns and scrapes to wounds.

ESSENTIAL REMEDY #44: WARTS—SAY GOOD-BYE
TO A BUMP WITH TEA TREE!

Bumps on the skin are not uncommon. The flesh-colored warts are benign growths, often on the hands, that are caused by a virus. You can go to a dermatologist and have them removed with a nitrogen spray. But sometimes it will require a second treatment. Or you can take the self-care route and see results, too.

What Scent-sational Oil Rx to Use: Dilute one drop of tea tree essential oil with one drop of apple cider vinegar and 2 drops of the carrier oil coconut oil. Apply the tea tree oil blend 2 times per day. It may take a few weeks for the DIY method to work.

Why You'll Feel Essentially Fine: Potent tea tree oil contains both antiseptic and antimicrobial properties. Paired with acetic acid–rich vinegar and anti-inflammatory coconut oil the solution should zap the wart(s). This method is less painful than the doctor's spray (or cutting!), and I can personally attest that vinegar does indeed do the trick. By compounding it with the essential oil and carrier oil, the odds are good that a wart may be history.

ESSENTIAL REMEDY #45: WRINKLES—ERASE AGING LINES!
GET THE LAVENDER CHILL.

In an age-obsessed society, lines on the face for both genders can be frowned upon. Wrinkles are more common if you're fair-skinned, have sun damage, or are past the age of seventy. If you don't want to head to a plastic surgeon (and I have not as yet), there is an essential oil remedy that may reduce the appearance of those lines.

What Scent-sational Oil Rx to Use: Fill an atomizer with one cup of water. Add 2 drops of lavender essential oil. Chill in the refrigerator. One cold spray on your face and neck. Repeat as needed.

Why You'll Essentially Feel Fine: Humidity and drinking plenty of water can give your facial skin a dewy look. Dehydration can make your skin look dull and lifeless. Lavender oil contains anti-inflammatory compounds that can soothe and moisturize dry skin.

Pairing lavender oil with H_2O may hydrate and rejuvenate your skin, providing a plumper and more radiant glow, minimizing the appearance of your life's lines like a roadmap.

SCENT-SATIONAL HEALING OILS SHORT & SWEET

Ailment	Oils & Scents	What It May Do
Acne	Tea tree oil	Heal your blemishes
Anxiety	Peppermint oil	Calms worry, uneasiness
Asthma Attack	Eucalyptus oil	Aid in breathing better
Athlete's foot	Peppermint oil	Soothes, heals
Boils	Vanilla oil	Fights infection, heals
Bruises	Rosemary oil	Heals inflammation, discoloring
Burns	Cedarwood	Soothes inflammation, stinging
Canker sores	Lavender oil	Soothes pain, swelling
Colds	Lavender oil	Lessens severity and recovery time
Cold sores	Lavender oil	Reduces pain, inflammation
Constipation	Cinnamon oil	Helps rev up regularity, relaxes intestines
Cough	Rosemary oil	Stops the tickle, scratchiness
Cuts	Tea tree oil	Fights inflammation, infection
Dizziness	Chamomile oil	Helps steadiness
Dry skin	Chamomile oil	Soothes redness, pain
Earache	Lavender oil and olive oil	Anti-inflammatory lessens throbbing
Fatigue	Lemon oil	Invigorates, lifts spirit
Fever	Chamomile oil	Helps regulate temperature
Fibromyalgia	Eucalyptus oil	Soothes aches and pains
Gum issues	Peppermint oil	Antimicrobial fights bacteria
Headaches	Chamomile oil	Quells throbbing
Heartburn	Chamomile oil and lemon or orange oil	Anti-inflammatory soothes the burning

(continued on p. 212)

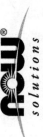

ESSENTIAL OIL	AROMA
Anise	Licorice-like, spicy
Atlas Cedar	Sweet, woodsy
Balsam Fir	Pleasant, woodsy
Basil	Warm, spicy
Bergamot	Sweet, fruity
Black Pepper	Dry, spicy, sharp
Camphor	Penetrating, medicinal
Carrot Seed	Earthy, woody, sweet
Cedarwood	Warm, woodsy, balsamic
Chamomile	Intense sweet, delightful
Cinnamon Bark	Warm, spicy
Cinnamon Cassia	Warm, spicy
Citronella	Pungent, musky, citrus-like
Clary Sage	Herbaceous, lavender-like
Clove	Warm, pungent
Cypress	Sweet balsamic, warm overtones of pine/juniper berry
Eucalyptus	Strong aromatic, camphoraceous
Eucalyptus Radiata	Fresh, camphorous, slightly sweet and minty
Frankincense	Mild camphor and citrus
Geranium	Subtly sweet, floral
Ginger	Spicy, warm
Grapefruit	Sweet, citrus
Hyssop	Camphor-like
Juniper Berry	Floral
Lavender	Floral
Lemon	Fresh lemon peel
Lemon Eucalyptus	Citronella-like with subtle floral undertones
Lemongrass	Strong, lemon-like
Lime	Fresh citrus lime
Marjoram	Camphoraceous, slightly medicinal
Myrrh	Musky, warm
Nutmeg	Spicy, nutty, soft, sweet aroma
Orange	Fresh, sweet orange peel
Oregano	Spicy, camphoraceous
Patchouli	Musky, earthy

MIXES WELL WITH	ATTRIBUTES
Cedarwood, Lime, Orange, Vanilla	Uplifting, balancing, comforting
Chamomile, Cypress, Eucalyptus, Sandalwood	Grounding, centering, balancing
Frankincense, Myrrh, Pine, Sandalwood Oil Blend	Empowering, balancing, strengthening
Bergamot, Citrus Oils, Hyssop	Uplifting, energizing, purifying
Lavender, Nutmeg, Citrus Oils	Lively, inspiring, uplifting
Geranium, Lavender, Frankincense, Citrus and Spice Oils	Warming, stimulating, focusing, cleansing
Cinnamon, Frankincense, Rosemary	Purifying, energizing, invigorating
Citrus Oils, Cedarwood, Lavender, Geranium	Soothing, rejuvenating, grounding
Cypress, Juniper, Rose, Sandalwood	Stress relief, strengthening, empowering
Bergamot, Grapefruit, Lemon, Tea Tree	Relaxing, calming, revitalizing
Clove, Nutmeg, Ginger, Vanilla	Warming, comforting, energizing
Clove, Ginger, Orange	Warming, stimulating, refreshing
Cedarwood, Lavender, Lemon, Lemongrass	Clarifying, freshening, purifying
Frankincense, Patchouli, Lime, Pine	Focusing, stimulating, balancing
Geranium, Ginger, Lavender, Lemon	Warming, soothing, comforting
Cedarwood, Citrus Oils, Clary Sage, Ylang Ylang	Balancing, clarifying, centering
Cedarwood, Cypress, Rosemary, Thyme	Revitalizing, invigorating, clarifying
Cinnamon, Rosemary, Tea Tree, Lavender, Clove	Repelling, clarifying, cleansing
Balsam Fir Needle, Myrrh, Orange, Sandalwood	Relaxing, focusing, centering
Clary Sage, Peppermint, Rose	Purifying, soothing, normalizing
Clove, Citrus Oils, Eucalyptus, Patchouli	Balancing, clarifying, stabilizing
Bergamot, Eucalyptus, Lemon, Thyme	Purifying, cheerful, uplifting
Clary Sage, Geranium, Rosemary, Sage	Clarifying, refreshing, purifying
Cypress, Eucalyptus, Rosemary, Sage	Restoring, empowering, balancing
Lemongrass, Peppermint, Marjoram, Tea Tree	Soothing, normalizing, balancing
Chamomile, Eucalyptus, Frankincense, Lavender	Refreshing, cheerful, uplifting
Geranium, Lavender, Cedarwood, Rosemary, Mint and Tree Oils	Refreshing, cleansing, stimulating
Citrus Oils, Geranium, Marjoram, Thyme	Purifying, stimulating, cleansing
Citrus Oils, Sage, Eucalyptus, Peppermint, Clove	Uplifting, refreshing, elating
Basil, Clary Sage, Rosemary, Thyme	Normalizing, comforting, warming
Frankincense, Patchouli, Sandalwood, Vanilla	Focusing, centering, meditative
Cinnamon, Clove, Orange, Vanilla	Energizing, stimulating, warming
Citrus Oils, Clove, Cinnamon, Nutmeg	Refreshing, uplifting, invigorating
Chamomile, Eucalyptus, Tea Tree, Spearmint	Purifying, comforting, invigorating
Cedarwood, Geranium, Lavender, Lemongrass	Romantic, soothing, stimulating

Pennyroyal	Fresh, minty-like
Peppermint	Fresh, strong mint
Pine	Balsamic, pine scent
Rosemary	Warm, camphoraceous
Sage	Warm, camphoraceous
Spearmint	Refreshing, minty
Spike Lavender	Herbaceous, floral, fresh
Tangerine	Pleasant, orange-like
Tea Tree	Potent, warm, spicy
Thyme, White	Pleasant, pungent
Wintergreen	Warm, sweet
Ylang Ylang Extra	Pleasant, floral

ESSENTIAL OIL BLENDS

Bottled Bouquet	Sweet, warm and floral with fresh citrus notes
Cheer Up Buttercup!	Citrus with light herbal
Clear the Air	Fresh mint
Frankincense 20%	Mild camphor and citrus
Good Morning Sunshine!	Citrus with slightly spicy undertone
Helichrysum	Sweet, herbaceous, earthy
Jasmine Absolute 7.5%	Warm, sweet floral
Jasmine Fragrance (Synthetic)	Warm, sweet floral
Lavender & Tea Tree	Soft, floral
Lemon & Eucalyptus	Citronella-like
Mental Focus	Minty citrus with wintergreen
Myrrh 20%	Mild, musky, warm aroma
Naturally Loveable	Sweet floral citrus
Nature's Shield	Sweet, invigorating, camphoraceous
Neroli 7.5%	Deep, floral aroma
Oil of Oregano 25%	Spicy, camphoraceous
Peace & Harmony	Minty floral herb
Peace, Love and Flowers	Sweet, floral
Peaceful Sleep	Floral citrus
Rose Absolute 5%	Pleasant rose
Sandalwood 14%	Subtle, floral, undertones of wood and fruit
Smiles for Miles	Citrus with light herbal
Vanilla	Sweet, warm

For information on Essential Oil Safety, go to nowfoods.com/eosafety.

Lemon, Eucalyptus, Lavender, Tea Tree	Repelling, stimulating
Eucalyptus, Juniper, Pine, Rosemary	Revitalizing, invigorating, cooling
Balsam Fir Needle, Cedarwood, Juniper Berry, Rosemary	Purifying, cleansing, refreshing
Bergamot, Lemongrass, Peppermint, Thyme	Purifying, uplifting
Citrus Oils, Hyssop, Lavender, Rosemary	Normalizing, balancing, soothing
Bergamot, Lavender, Lime, Rosemary	Cooling, invigorating, stimulating
Florals, Pine, Tea Tree, Balsam Fir Needle	Clarifying, balancing, comforting
Cinnamon, Citrus Oils, Nutmeg, Vanilla	Cheerful, inspiring, invigorating
Basil, Cypress, Eucalyptus, Lemon, Lavender, Thyme	Cleansing, purifying, renewing
Basil, Lavender, Lemon, Marjoram	Uplifting, empowering, clarifying
Eucalyptus, Lemon, Peppermint, Tangerine	Stimulating, refreshing, uplifting
Citrus Oils, Clove, Jasmine, Patchouli, Rose	Soothing, romantic, comforting

Pre-blended and ready for use	Romantic, balancing, calming
Pre-blended and ready for use	Uplifting, refreshing, energizing
Pre-blended and ready for use	Purifying, cleansing, refreshing
Balsam Fir Needle, Myrrh, Orange, Sandalwood	Relaxing, focusing, centering
Pre-blended and ready for use	Energizing, focusing, soothing
Lavender, Bergamot, Rose, Cypress	Soothing, rejuvenating, stimulating
Citrus Oils, Ylang Ylang, Vanilla, Rose	Romantic, relaxing, calming
Citrus Oils, Clove, Ginger, Ylang Ylang	Romantic, relaxing, calming
Lavender, Eucalyptus, Rose Absolute	Renewing, cleansing, stimulating
Thyme, Lavender, Rosemary, Lemon	Clarifying, cleansing, invigorating
Pre-blended and ready for use	Balancing, centering, focusing
Frankincense, Patchouli, Sandalwood Oil Blend	Focusing, grounding, meditative
Pre-blended and ready for use	Romantic, comforting, calming
Pre-blended and ready for use	Uplifting, energizing, freshening and cleansing
Citrus Oils, Chamomile, Patchouli, Ylang Ylang	Calming, soothing, centering
Chamomile, Eucalyptus, Tea Tree, Spearmint	Purifying, comforting, invigorating
Pre-blended and ready for use	Centering, calming, balancing
Pre-blended and ready for use	Calming, soothing, uplifting
Pre-blended and ready for use	Calming, relaxing, soothing
Bergamot, Jasmine, Lavender, Lemon, Sandalwood	Romantic, uplifting, comforting
Citrus Oils, Frankincense, Jasmine, Vanilla, Lavender	Grounding, focusing, balancing
Pre-blended and ready for use	Uplifting, refreshing, energizing
Citrus Oils, Jasmine, Rose, Sandalwood, Ylang Ylang	Comforting, relaxing, nurturing

SCENT-SATIONAL HEALING OILS SHORT & SWEET (cont.)

Ailment	Oils & Scents	What It May Do
Hemorrhoids	Chamomile oil	Lessens inflammation, itching
Hypochondria	Rose oil	Helps calm nerves, worry
Inattentive	Lemon oil	Triggers focus, mental energy
Insect bites	Peppermint oil	Soothes inflammation, redness
Insomnia	Geranium oil	Relaxes, calms nerves
Irritable bowel syndrome	Peppermint oil	Regulates digestive system
Jet lag	Orange oil	Boosts mental, physical alertness
Low libido	Sandalwood	Boosts confidence, well-being
Menopausal hot flashes	Peppermint oil	Helps to cool down
Migraine	Peppermint oil	Rids throbbing, pain, nausea
Panic attack	Sandalwood oil and chamomile oil	Helps to calm, center attention
PMS Cramps	Peppermint oil	Soothes muscle pain
Poison oak/ivy	Lavender oil	Stops itch, stinging
Seasonal Affective Disorder	Vanilla Oil	Vanillin calms and and grounds you
Sinusitis	Eucalyptus oil	Aids in congestion
Sore throat	Lemon oil	Soothes irritation, burning
Sprains	Eucalyptus oil	Relieves aches and pains
Stress	Vanilla oil	Calms and centers
Tongue burn	Lavender oil	Anti-inflammatory heals the swelling, redness
Toothache	Clove oil	Numbs pain
Universal E.R. conditions	Lavender oil	Soothes body, mind, and spirit with its calming and antibacteria and anti-inflammatory compounds
Warts	Peppermint oil	Shrinks bumps
Wrinkles	Lavender	Help in smoothing skin

PART 5

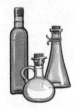

AROMAMANIA

Beautifying Oils

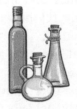

The earth laughs in flowers.
—RALPH WALDO EMERSON

The snowy drive for the Reno book event that I shared in the last chapter was no spa day. However, a past trip to Victoria, Canada, did include aromatherapy—and it was an unforgettable treat for a long trek. To unwind on the first day in a foreign land, I treated myself to an aromatic manicure, including a hand massage with a lotion infused with peppermint essential oil. I was instantly invigorated. The familiar fragrance took me home. It reminded me of the minty oil manicure I had enjoyed at a spa close to my home in northern California. That empty feeling of disconnectedness when in another country is unsettling. I can tell you, though, a familiar aroma, like a recognizable song, is a lifeline to relaxation. Essential oils can make you feel calmer. I felt safe, like I do when I'm in my cabin with the scent of pine trees and a diffuser in the kitchen, my favorite citrus oil permeating the autumn air. Even though I was all alone in a big foreign city, surrounded by skyscrapers and strangers, the recognizable peppermint essential oil on my hands felt like meeting and hugging a friend.

SPA'D WITH ESSENTIAL OILS

Luxury spas offer an array of essential oils in their beauty treatment menu. In my twenties and thirties, health spas I went to offered extra perks, such as massages, saunas, and steams. And aromatherapy and essential oils, including eucalyptus and citrus scents, were used to enhance the scene. In my forties, I'd interview spa directors from Canyon Ranch in Arizona and New York, and aromatherapy once again greeted me as the beauty treatment wizards would tantalize me with their latest lineup for their spa-goers. And now, living in a resort town, I do regularly swim and use the hot tub at a hotel resort; sometimes I can smell an essential oil aroma permeating the air while a spa guest is getting pampered in the treatment rooms.

Here, take a peek at some popular spa treatments that include aromatherapy and essential oils for mind, body, and spiritual benefits.

Facials: There are umpteen aromatherapy facials available to you at spas. Essential oils are selected for your specific needs, whether it is for exfoliating and smoothing to getting a rosy glow or moisturizing and hydrating for anti-aging benefits.

Body Scrub: Getting a head-to-toe treatment is similar to a facial, but your total body is pampered. The technician will select a custom-tailored essential oil blend for your body and its needs. It could be for relaxing, rejuvenating, or even to counteract cellulite.

Body Skin Wrap: This spa treatment is less interactive than a scrub. Once your body is wrapped up like a mummy, you'll let the essential oils blend do the work instead of a hands-on type scrub. It, too, can offer many therapeutic benefits.

Hydrotherapy: Hot, bubbly water can be invigorating and relaxing. Hydrotherapy, aka a tub with jet-powered bubbles, can help increase your blood circulation to aid in relaxing tense muscles from anxiety, stress, or overexertion in play or work.

Zesty Lemon Honey Gommage

Here's a treatment you can try at home. This lemon honey gommage cream, which is simply a scrub, can gently exfoliate the face and/or body and give your skin a radiant glow. It's a super blend with citrus, floral, and herbal essential oils to use time after time, for getting your *Stella's Groove* mojo back and look radiant—at any age.

*4 tablespoons bentonite or kaolin clay**
3 tablespoons mineral water
*¼ teaspoon powdered lemon balm herb**
1 tablespoon honey
3 drops bergamot essential oil
2 drops rosemary essential oil
1 drop lavender essential oil

In a glass or rubber bowl, mix bentonite clay and water until creamy in texture. Add lemon balm and honey until completely blended. Slowly stir in bergamot, rosemary, and lavender essential oils until all ingredients are combined. It may be necessary to add more bentonite clay. Apply with clean fingertips to clean skin. Leave on for 10 minutes or until dry. Remove in short "rolling" motions until completely removed from skin. Rinse well and apply appropriate moisturizer. Store unused mixture in a covered container, away from direct sunlight and heat to preserve its optimum quality for up to one week.

*Items are available in most health food stores or herb shops or by going online.

Benefits: Exfoliating and antibacterial. Will make skin clean and polished, soft and smooth.

(Courtesy: National Honey Board)

THE QUINTESSENTIAL
INTERVIEW WITH A LUXURY SPA DIRECTOR

I can tell you honestly that using at home essential oil treatments are super, but getting pampered at a spa by yourself, with friends, or a partner is simply sublime. Welcome to Cal-a-Vie Health Spa and Resort. You're now entering an impressive spa located in northern San Diego County, California. The estate resembles a breathtaking French village. Cal-a-Vie offers spa cuisine and European-style beauty and spa treatments. In an exclusive interview, I asked the savvy spa director about the usage of essential oils and aromatherapy for benefits to the health and well-being of guests at Cal-a-Vie.

Q: *I have three Vinotherapie aromatic beauty body items, a cream, gel, and lotion, which are made from wine grape seed, skin, and pulp from your vineyard—and essential oils, including citrus oil like neroli and tangerine. Is there a garden on the premises that has plants used for essential oils in your spa's beauty treatments?*

A: We have beautiful gardens on our property, but Body Bliss provides our essential oils. We do use many of the herbs and flowers in several of our treatments. We do a Poultice Massage that incorporates chamomile, lavender, and sage in the poultice that we source here from the property.

Q: *You had me at lavender, my favorite herb and essential oil. Did you say lavender fields?*

A: We do have an expansive lavender field on the property and several lavender plants sprinkled throughout the land. It smells heavenly in the springtime.

Q: *Essential oil–infused body items are believed to promote smooth, healthy, youthful skin. How does it do this?*

A: Amyris and lavender oils help heal skin irritations and can be used for all skin types. They can calm down stressed skin. Chamomile can treat a variety of skin conditions, which include acne, eczema, inflammation, rosacea, and sensitive skin. Neroli and tangerine are wonderful essential oils used to treat aging and mature skin.

Q: *Which type of massage treatments include essential oils?*

A: We use our essential oils in our Aromatic Awakening massage. We take our guests on a sensory journey and let them choose the oil that calls to them. Very often, you choose what your body needs.

Q: *I enjoyed a spa hydrotherapy session that included honey and orange essential oil—it was an unforgettable experience because I felt like a princess; afterword my skin was like silk to touch. What type of bubbling water healing oil pleasures does your spa offer?*

A: We offer five different oil blends. The most popular is Restore; it has lemon, rose, and ylang-ylang to bring balance and peace. Six months ago, we had a woman come in and she had just finished her last round of chemo. She was very emotional. She shared that she chose Love [which includes a few of my top 20 essential oil picks: jasmine, sandalwood, and vanilla] because it was now time to heal herself with self-love.

She came out from the treatment radiating with smiles and said that she had not felt that good in a long time. We made a little gift basket for her and included the same products we used in her treatment so she could continue with the bathing ritual at home.

Q: *Scrub therapy. You use blue chamomile and lavender. This blend has calmed me already. Is there a big demand for the blend treatment?*

A: Yes. Our scrub therapy is done in our shower room and is a full body treatment. Blue chamomile is used for calming and soothing skin and assists with inflammation. It is incredibly relaxing and leaves the skin feeling so smooth and hydrated.

Q: *And your body wrap therapy uses a honey lavender blend. Is the lavender from the lavender essential oil?*

A: Yes, it is. This wrap begins with a luxurious scrub to exfoliate and improve circulation. Next, warmed honey will be drizzled on your body before you are cocooned in a warming blanket to indulge in the luscious goodness of this wrap. After showering, you will receive an application of a lavender-infused lotion.

Q: *Is it rewarding to see your guests enjoy the world of essential oils in these spa treatments?*

A: We had a guest that had traveled here from France. She was exhausted and congested. She came out of the treatment so relaxed from being massaged with lavender and her therapist did some inhalation breathing. I have vast experience with essential oils, and it is so rewarding for me to actually see the benefits these oils have on our guests.

DIY BEAUTY-UP TIPS AND RECIPES

Wherever you are, at a luxury spa or away on a trip, essential oils are, well, you know, beautifying, comforting, and can help you feel right at home. My top 20 essential oil picks are in this chapter and they are also accompanied by other essential oils for the ultimate beautifying effect. You don't have to whisk away on a jet plane to a posh resort to get spa'd and achieve the scent-sation of feeling and looking your best. I've chosen some common essential oil combos that will help you get a beauty treatment to love. And you'll find your own blends that may be even a better fit for you and your body. Here, these easy-to-make potions will get you on the fragrant essential path to beauty with essential oils at home.

SOFT FACE

Essential oils offer many benefits for different skin types, which can change with climate, hormones, and age. These essential oils may already be included in the ingredients of the skin products you use or you can add them into your skin care regime, depending on your specific needs and time of year. When I was in my twenties, I coped with oily and dry skin. These days, my skin can be dry, especially during the wintertime, and due to the age factor. I use an unscented moisturizer with SPF 30 for sensitive skin. I tried adding a tiny toothpick amount of lavender into the lotion and put it on my wrist for a patch test. No problems and a nice touch!

Dry skin: Lavender and rose.
Normal skin: Geranium and rose.
Oily skin: Lemon and tea tree.

Try a Mediterranean Facial: Resort spas offer facials but you can also do it yourself. Simply steam your face over a large pot of hot water infused with 1 drop of an essential oil noted for your skin type for about 10 minutes. Rinse with cool water and pat dry. Enjoy the rosy glow.

SILKY BODY

A bath is not only relaxing and rejuvenating, paired with essential oils it can offer more perks. Kobashi's Lynda Ballard recommends, "Dilute up to six drops of an essential oil into a bath or soap base. Add to the water." Then, you can sit back, relax, and simply enjoy the aromatic water. "Orange and geranium are a pleasant balancing blend. Rosemary and lavender can be invigorating. The oils are all synergistic and work well when combined. These combinations are endless."

Smooth Hands

Before you get a manicure try a hand balm to get your hands looking smooth.

LAVENDER HAND BALM

1½ ounces jojoba oil
3 ounces jojoba oil
3 ounces shea butter (additional, if needed)
1½ ounces beeswax beads
½ teaspoon lavender essential oil
¼ teaspoon lemon essential oil

In a Pyrex measuring cup, combine jojoba, shea butter, and beeswax. Set in a pan of simmering water (water should reach ¼ of the way up the side of the Pyrex cup). Stir until wax is completely melted. Remove from heat and stir in lavender and lemon oils. Pour into a wide-mouth, half-pint (8-ounce) jar and cool overnight.
Note: This recipe makes a firm balm. For a softer salve,

add up to 2 more tablespoons jojoba oil. Store in re-frigerator.

Makes about 6 ounces.

(Courtesy: LorAnn Oils)

CROWNING GLORY

Store-bought hair products, from shampoos to conditioners, vary for specific needs. For instance, I use a volumizing, conditioning shampoo for fine hair. By adding lavender to it, I get a pleasant floral scent for my long, curly locks. You can try it, too. Simply add 1 drop of an essential oil to 12 ounces of your shampoo or conditioner, depend-ing on your hair type for best results.

Dry hair: Lavender or rosemary.
Normal hair: Chamomile or lavender.
Oily hair: Patchouli or tea tree.

Dry Hair Recipe

Living in the mountains without a lot of humidity leaves my long hair dry. I love this essential oil recipe that can work wherever you live.

15 mL jojoba oil
10 drops sandalwood essential oil
10 drops lavender essential oil
10 drops everlast essential oil [Helichrysum (everlast)
    oils are from Corsica; from flower tops]

Combine all the ingredients and apply to hair. This formula is best left on for 20 minutes and then washed out with a gentle shampoo.

(Courtesy: Monika Haas, Director of Pacific Institute of Aromatherapy)

Essentially Beautifying Lemon Drop Body Wash

❖ ❖ ❖

This citrus-scented body wash with lemon essential oil is simple but one to share for its basic ingredients and optimum results. After living in the mountains for two decades, I've tried to adapt to the lack of humidity and dry air, which can wreak havoc on your skin. This wash is soothing and an energizing super starter to keep your body softer and smoother (at any age).

But note, I do have all-natural essential oils–based body wash brands in my shower, too. These provide more complex washes with essential oil blends, including vanilla and lavender essential oils. Starting simple and adding a bit more is essential if you live in a dry climate and do not want dry skin.

2 cups unscented castile soap
2 cups honey
½ cup lemon juice
3–4 drops lemon essential oil

Combine all the ingredients into a bottle and shake. Use with a sponge or washcloth, massage desired amount over entire body and rinse. Store in shower. Use daily.

Yield: 1 bottle.

(Courtesy: National Honey Board)

You've got the idea about how essential oils and aromatherapy can be a beautifying experience, but why stop here? I adore having my home earthy and cozy. Enter essential oils and aromatherapy. Plant therapy can help you to enhance your body, mind, spirit—and household! Discover in the next chapter how nature's scents can spruce up your environment, room by room, indoors or out.

SCENT-SATIONAL HEALING OILS SHORT & SWEET

✓ If you're looking to spa-beautify your body and well-being, antioxidant-rich essential oils are for you. Yes, they can help you look your best, rejuvenate, and/or relax your body . . .

✓ And whether you go to a spa or use essential oils at home, you can achieve results from the oils . . .

✓ And aromatic treatments enhance therapeutic body benefits of a massage or hydrotherapy treatment.

✓ Essential oils, like stimulating peppermint and calming lavender, can rejuvenate and relax. Indeed, healing oils can create inner and outer beauty!

✓ Fragrant healing essential oils add a special touch to any beauty treatment.

✓ Essential oils often include antibacterial and anti-inflammatory compounds that can be used on your body for soothing and smoothing beautifying benefits and have been appreciated since the beginning of time.

Essential Oils for a
Healthy Household

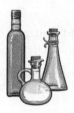

*Your oils have a pleasing fragrance. Your name is
like purified oil.*
—SONG OF SOLOMON 1:3

Ah, nature's garden . . . After a decade of living at Lake Tahoe, I noticed the scent of vacation homeowners seemed to be more striking
and easily identifiable. One summer thanks to my keen sense of smell,
the aroma of barbecue meat, suntan lotion, and alcohol at noon alerted
me to their presence. Instead of complaining, I created a scented garden indoors and outdoors.

I put basil and rosemary potted plants in the sun-filled windowsills
in the kitchen and dining room. A cumbersome vaporizer was stacked
on a book shelf in the dining room/study—but the cat jumped up and
it came tumbling down. I made a summertime potpourri full of floral

oils (but they were two decades old), so the kitchen didn't smell like flowers. Sadly, the plants wilted, leaf by leaf. My fantasy of having a *Lady Chatterley's Lover*–type indoor aromatic garden turned into a spooky plant graveyard disaster.

ZEN WAYS TO FRESH AIR

There are limitless ways to put aromatherapy to work in your home. To add essential oils into your environment at home for medicinal, therapeutic, spiritual, and cosmetic benefits, here's some things you can do to get yourself started.

Aromatic Sprays—spritz and sniff: A bottle that contains your favorite essential oil(s) and water. Mist it anywhere—and feel a boost in your mood with lemon oil, or calm nerves calm with sandalwood. Simply, choose your oil of choice and take charge of the air around you.

Aromatic Pottery Diffusers: They work as a slow diffusion of essential oil. To scent a room put a couple of drops of an essential oil in a pottery diffuser. I have a small navy blue–colored pot with a cork top, which is a sentimental gift from an arts fair in Berkeley, California. It is on top of a ledge in the bathroom (away from companion animals' reach). They make aromatherapy easy to take with you everywhere, whether it be at work, traveling, or in the comfort of your home.

Humidifier Diffuser: An easy breezy way to disperse oil in the air is by using this electric diffuser. It's a device that disperses a mist of pure essential oil and water in the air. This device can vary in price, from $16 to $200 or more. I purchased a small, popular device available online. The diffuser humidifier with mist mode has seven color LED lights, which change as the essential oil and water mix mists the air.

Steam Vaporizers: Like the electric humidifier, these are another way to inhale essential oils. I have one because the air is so dry where I live. But note, some devices are not to be used with essential oils because they are too potent and can erode the plastic of the humidifier.

ESSENTIAL OILS FOR YOUR HOME—ROOM BY ROOM

During college I cleaned homes as a source of income. The downside was using the smelly chemical cleaning products. Usually, I was left home alone to do chores. To prevent boredom, I enjoyed cleaning the house, task by task, instead of room by room.

If I were to go back in time, I'd push more for natural cleaners infused with essential oils. Here, take a look at a day's work from my past with a scented fix.

BATHROOMS

I always began with the bathrooms, which usually included three or more in homes that were more than two thousand square feet. If there were stains, I'd let the cleaning agents soak before scrubbing.

Sinks, Toilets, Shower/Tub: Instead of a strong Ajax-type cleaner, making your own, like my recipe, can work well. Mix 1 cup of baking soda with ½ cup white vinegar and 2 drops of a citrus essential oil, like lemon or orange. Both the vinegar and oils have antibacterial compounds in them, and the baking soda is abrasive to clean.

Countertops: Get your house clean and fresh with this DIY cleaning solution.

All-Natural Cleaning Solution

This bathroom/house cleaner features lemon and tea tree essential oils for disinfecting muscle.

¼ cup white vinegar
1 cup water
12 drops lemon essential oil
8 drops tea tree essential oil
6 drops eucalyptus essential oil

Mix together all ingredients in a spray bottle. Shake before using to distribute oils. Avoid use on natural stone and wood.

(Courtesy: LorAnn Oils)

BEDROOMS

The sleeping areas, often four or more rooms, entailed changing beds, dusting, and vacuuming.

Vacuuming the Floor/Carpet: Customize with your favorite essential oils to make a scent you love.

Natural Carpet & All-Purpose Deodorizer
❖ ❖ ❖

Try mixing with lavender, orange, or tangerine essential oils for a refreshing blend.

1 cup baking soda
30 drops natural essential oils of your choice

In a glass jar with a lid, combine and shake together baking soda and essential oils until oils are well dispersed. To freshen carpets, sprinkle liberally over carpets or rugs. Allow to sit for at least 30 minutes. Vacuum well.

(Courtesy: LorAnn Oils)

Get Rid of Moths! One winter day, I noticed tiny holes in my favorite sweaters and T-shirts. I cleaned out my bedroom drawers and all my clothes closets. I didn't find any bugs but wanted to do something to prevent another occurrence. That's when I went to the hardware store and purchased an Armageddon survivor's supply of cedarwood. Cedarwood blocks, balls, and hangar blocks remain in my closets and drawers to this day. The moth-repellant wood blocks are natural instead of toxic like sprays to keep bugs away. Once the scent dissipates, instead of buying new cedarwood products, I revive them. First, I wipe each piece of wood with a clean cloth followed by a piece of sandpaper. Then, with another cloth I rub a few drops of cedarwood essential oil on each square. I let the cedar blocks dry in the sun for one day. The rich balsamic scent is back. It's eco-friendly without using toxic sprays, which is healthier for our planet, me, and my family.

LIVING/DINING ROOM

These rooms often had more traffic from family and friends, so extra care for furniture, dusting, and vacuuming was next in line.

Restoring Furniture: If you have a favorite leather sofa, lemon essential oil can help it look almost new. Use a drop or two on the leather and wipe. But note, be careful! One afternoon after reading that I could use lemon essential oil on leather scratches, I put it to work. After two drops rubbed with a dry cloth on the arm of the love seat, I was amazed! I couldn't see the surface scratches. At all. I put more drops of oil on the seats. I ended up using more than a dozen drops of the lemon oil. Soon, the scent was too potent and permeated throughout the living room. I was alarmed. Turning on the ceiling fan and two floor fans wasn't enough ventilation. I opened all the windows, and the front door. For safety's sake, I put the cat in a crate, the dog on a leash, and escaped outdoors for an hour.

I flushed my nose with bottled water because it burned inside. My heart rate was probably over 100. I fantasized about calling 9-1-1.

"Ma'am, what is your emergency?"

I would answer, "A toxic lemon essential oil spill."

"Excuse me?"

I decided against the call. Instead of getting first responders at my home, I drank plenty of water and gave water to my dog. I started to calm down after the lemon oil event. Yes, the powerful lemon oil worked to beautify my couch, but I paid the price. Remember, less is more.

KITCHEN

I always saved the kitchen for last because it was the most challenging. This room is more detailed with countertops, the oven, outside appliances, sink, silverware, dusting, and vacuuming.

Countertops: Using a few drops of lemon essential oil with water in a spray bottle is a good disinfectant. Lemon oil also provides a refreshing aroma. It is known for its antimicrobial properties, which can halt bacteria.

Oven Cleaner: Scrubbing ovens is one job I enjoyed. It is a challenge to turn a greasy mess into a clean and shiny appliance. I didn't mind the elbow grease needed for this dirty task, but the chemical cleaners were not eco-friendly. I wish I'd had a green spray cleaner, but the homeowners did not. These days, when I clean the stovetop and oven I turn to natural cleaners. This recipe, created just for me and you is a godsend.

All-Natural Oven Cleaner Recipe

½ cup hot water
½ cup white distilled vinegar
1 tablespoon Sal-Suds (optional but recommended)
30 drops lemon essential oil
10 drops thyme essential oil

Mix all ingredients in a spray bottle. Spray the inside of the oven and allow it to set for 5 minutes. Spray the inside of the oven once more and then wipe out with a paper towel or sponge. Gloves are recommended.

(Courtesy: Plant Therapy)

Stainless Steel Polish: I didn't like wiping down toasters, dishwashers, and refrigerators with Windex or another all-purpose cleaner with ingredients I couldn't pronounce. Try this!

Stainless Steel Polish Recipe

❖ ❖ ❖

½ cup jojoba oil
20 drops lemon essential oil
20 drops pine essential oil

Mix all ingredients in a spray bottle. Spray on stainless steel appliances and allow it to set for a minute. Buff it off with a microfiber cloth.

(Courtesy: Plant Therapy)

KEEP IT GREEN OUTDOORS

Wash the Windows: When I washed windows, I preferred using vinegar and water. The aroma was fine but it lacked a special scent. These days, it's all-natural window cleaner with essential oils included.

Window Cleaner

❖ ❖ ❖

1 cup vinegar [I use Heinz white vinegar]
1 cup water
20 drops lavender
10 drops peppermint

Mix all ingredients in a spray bottle. Spray on window and wipe with microfiber cloth.

(Courtesy: Plant Therapy)

Rid of Ants: Ants can be found inside the home as well as outdoors. One time my job was to clean a friend's home when he was away on a business trip. Once I arrived on the back porch, dozens of ants were everywhere, thanks to his son's beer party and leftover cans. Not wanting to use a toxic spray, I was left with soap, water, and elbow grease for what seemed like an eternity with the killer ants. It's important to find the source, as I did.

But now, I have discovered a better way to be the ant terminator by turning to an effective essential oil for help. Try this!

Peppermint Oil Natural Bug Repellant

❖ ❖ ❖

2 cups water
10–15 drops peppermint essential oil

Combine water and peppermint oil in a spray bottle. Shake bottle before use and spray solution around entry spots such as windowsills and door frames, or places where insects may hide. The strong odor acts as a repellant.

(Courtesy: LorAnn Oils)

ESSENTIAL OILS CRAZE

So, I'm sure you're wondering just how common essential oils are in American households. What is the breakdown of how they are used by people like you and me? The results are surprising and may change a bit as essential oils grow more popular in the mainstream. But this is a working guide gleaned from a variety of aromatherapy go-to experts to give you an idea of the breakdown of oils and how they are used by people. Food and flavors, 50 percent; fragrance and medicinal and healing uses, 40 percent; cleaning products and aromatherapy, fall into the lowest tier.

In the media, from magazines to the Internet, you'll discover a buzz continues year after year on what's new in essential oils and aromatherapy. Medical studies around the globe pop up continually on which essential oils can help lower the risk of a variety of health issues from minor ailments to life-threatening diseases. Celebs, from Demi Moore to Gwen Paltrow, popular health and women's magazines, like *Marie Claire, Allure,* and *First for Women,* run stories on the powers of healing oils, which are touted to be in demand as cancer fighters, fat fighters, and age fighters.

Dr. Mehmet Oz, the renowned TV doctor, discusses the connection of essential oils and health. In one of his programs he touts a variety of oils, including lavender and peppermint, two of the most popular essential oils—and olive oil, my favorite carrier oil.

But the thrill of essential oils doesn't stop there. According to research companies who seek out trends, essential oils and aromatherapy are here to stay and are gaining popularity.

That's right. Healing oils are being used in hospitals and the workplace and inside homes, like yours and mine. More than three-fourths of Americans will use essentials oils for scent in their households by 2020. We're going to see more usage of aromatherapy and healing oils for DIY health ailments, lowering the risk of depression, heart disease, obesity, and even cancer. Simply do an online search for the words "essential oil trends," and you'll continue to see a lot of trend forecasts from companies who predict real crazes for the future. Yes, essential oils are here and finding your favorites has been made easier than ever!

Pacific Institute of Aromatherapy's Kurt Schnaubelt has also noticed the surge of interest in essential oils and aromatherapy. He points out, "Aromatherapy is finding broader acceptance." He gives the credit to the efforts of the large multilevel marketing companies. "As more people try essential oils," adds Dr. Schnaubelt, "they inadvertently become subject to the physiological benefits . . . and gravitate back to them."

There are more essential oil companies in the twenty-first century in contrast to the twentieth century when aromatherapy was a wave in the holistic industry. But now, the noise of essential oils is like a scented tsunami. (Refer to the Essential Oils Resources in the back of the book for some popular brand names, devices, and accessories for all your essential oil and aromatherapy needs.)

SCENTED OIL CANDLES FOR HEALING

Not only can essential oils provide a warm and fuzzy feeling—scented candles infused with essential oils are something to write home about, too. Candle company manufacturers will tell you candles can be traced back to ancient Egypt, where tombs reveal carvings of candles. In the 1800s, candles were used for light to see. And in the 1900s, we used candles for ambience during dining and emergencies such as power outages. In the twenty-first century, you, like me, may use a variety of candles, in different sizes, colors, and types for a variety of reasons.

Some essential oils can be used in aromatherapy blends for candles, which can be soothing. Aromatherapy candles will enhance your well-being differently, depending on your chosen blends. Take a look at which candles can be used in your home for a myriad of benefits.

Colds and Congestion: If you're feeling under the weather with a cold or flu bug, you know how to use healing oils to help feel better and recover. I have a white candle in the bathroom that has a blend of a variety of essential oils, including vanilla. (Best candles: eucalyptus, lavender, marjoram, and peppermint.)

Fatigue and Low Mood: During hectic holidays, seasonal change, or life's events, we can and do sometimes begin to feel tired and a bit down. In the dining room, I have a light green mint candle that I have used when I'm cooking to give me an energy boost. (Best candles: basil, geranium, peppermint, and rosemary.)

Rest and Relaxation: In a busy world we often get caught up in trying to do it all. This is why people take vacations—to rejuvenate their mind and body. But turning to a scented candle can feel like a mini escape. In my bedroom, I have calming vanilla-scented candles for when power outages happen during winter snowstorms and summer thunderstorms. (Best candles: geranium, lavender, patchouli, and ylang-ylang.)

Stress and Tension: Feeling stressed out or tense due to life's ups and downs in the workplace and home? Light a calming candle and take a bath or maybe lie down in the bedroom with a good book. This can help you decompress and enjoy the moment. In the living room I keep an assortment of vanilla candles on the fireplace mantel. Pair this calming scent with one of the relaxing activities listed above and unwind. (Best candles: chamomile, jasmine, juniper, and melissa.)

A Natural Mom and Essential Oils

You'll discover as I did, that some gentle essential oils are used for children and companion animals. Lynda Ballard of Kobashi Ltd. gives a real-life peek at how she has put to work essential oils for her family. Read on and take in her words of wisdom with essential oil and the family . . .

Babies: As new parents here in the UK, we are given a welcome pack containing samples of well-known commercial baby care products. None of these contained anything we would wish to use on ourselves let alone a new baby. So as our journey with Lily began, we started adding to the baby products. A baby lotion with lavender and chamomile, and a baby bath and oil. I can honestly say she never suffered any sort of nappy rash.

Ants: While on a family holiday in Minorca, the apartment we were staying in was visited daily by tiny ants. They came in through small cracks in the walls and around the windows. The owner of the apartment was well aware of the problem but said it was a common experience on the island. They had left us with a large aerosol spray bottle of insecticide. We never use any of these sprays as we don't like killing things and also know how harmful these toxic chemicals are to us as human beings. So once again out came our essential oils. We put down a few drops of lemon and cinnamon first thing in the morning and last thing at night. This confuses the ant's sense of smell, and without this they are not able to follow their scent trails. This did the trick and the added bonus was that the whole apartment smelled wonderful.

Cats: Orange oil is also used a lot in our house. We inherited two beautiful Bengal cats when their owner passed away. They are both neutered males but still felt the need to mark as much territory in order to establish themselves in their new homes, which of course they had to share with us! After cleaning the sprayed area with a mixture of eucalyptus, tea tree, and lavender diluted in our soap base, I sprinkled orange oil and this has certainly stopped any repeated spraying. Both cats have now thankfully settled down. [Author's note: I tried this remedy for my dog who marked one area spot on an oriental rug I like. No more accidents. My theory is the essential oil fragrance covered up his scent. Since it did its job, I stopped using the essential oil spray.]

Essential Oils for Kids and Pets

Using essential oils for infants and toddlers and companion animals is a controversial topic. I went to aromatherapy guru, Kurt Schnaubelt. He says, "Using essential oils with children is difficult because despite low or no toxicity, some oils simply create such strong sensory impact that it throws children off and leads to unpredictable reactions."

I agree with Dr. Schnaubelt. Now, I would love to put 1 drop of calming lavender essential oil behind the ears of my excitable Australian shepherd, especially during the busy tourist season, but I feel more at ease putting a dab of lavender oil on my wrist so I can cope better with his barking at wayward dogs, car doors slamming, concerts, and fireworks. Or perhaps in the future I can give essential oil gift baskets to vacation homeowners so they can chill and tune out the "woof, woof, woof."

Since the jury is still out on the safety of using essential oils on human children and fur children, I will not use any essential oil products on my dog or cat. But note, there are essential oil lines for both children and pets that you can find online. Before using any essential oils for your kids or fur children, please consult with your doctor and/or veterinarian for safety's sake.

Naturally Cleansing
Garden Salad with Lavender Oil Dressing

❖ ❖ ❖

Using essential oils helps you to eat more of nature's foods, including fresh salads. In my college days, salad bars were my favorite meal when going to restaurants. I was able to eat a larger variety of fruits and vegetables. Since then, I've learned adding essential oils to a dressing adds flavor and aroma. This recipe is simple but if you're not a salad person, you may convert to one. When the weather's nice, a garden salad in the great outdoors will allow you to enjoy plant therapy all the more. Can you smell the lavender?

2 cups kale and cabbage mix, chopped
¼ cup walnuts, chopped
¼ cup cranberries, dried

DRESSING

2 tablespoons herbal vinegar
½ clove garlic, minced
1 teaspoon honey
1 teaspoon rosemary, fresh, chopped
1 drop lavender essential oil
1 drop lemon essential oil
¼ cup extra virgin olive oil

In a bowl, combine kale mix, nuts, and berries. Set aside. In another bowl, mix vinegar, garlic, honey, rosemary, and essential oils with olive oil. Drizzle on top of salad.

Serves 2.

It's time. The exciting part of this book has arrived. You know that essential oils can be used in foods, and I've teased you with some food recipes. But you may not know how they can be used in a wide variety of dishes. And now, the grand recipes finale is here. Let's get cooking by mixing and matching essential oils with nutritious foods. But first, there are some essential details and a sample diet plan you'll want to view to build your confidence before you hit the kitchen and enjoy the culinary essential oils.

SCENT-SATIONAL HEALING OILS SHORT & SWEET

✓ If you have chemical sensitivities inside and outside your home, find eco-friendly products that include essential oils and/or use DIY essential oil recipes as a healthful alternative to harsh cleaners.

✓ It's never too early to introduce your kids to essential oils. Start s-l-o-w-l-y and proceed with caution using kid-friendly healing oils.

✓ There are reputable essential oil companies that offer kid-friendly and pet-friendly essential oils. But note, contact your vet or health-care practitioner before using any oil on a two-legger or four-legger.

✓ Essential oils, thanks to their aromatic healing gifts, can be used for arts and crafts in the household and are healthy in contrast to using chemical-laden items.

PART 6

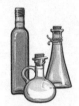

EDIBLE ESSENTIAL FOOD RECIPES

The Joy of Cooking with Edible Oils

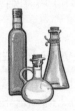

I have smelt all the aromas there are in the fragrant kitchen they call Earth, and what we can enjoy in this life. I surely have enjoyed just like a Lord!
—HEINRICH HEINE

One summer night after tending to my mountain-style garden with some landscaping, a deck, and hardy cactus potted plants . . . something was missing. I was craving a cold treat to pair with iced tea. I found an unopened large container of vanilla gelato. But it was mint chocolate chip I wanted. The thought of going out into the town filled with tourists was not an option. So I opened the kitchen pantry and was pleasantly surprised, like a kid finding an unwrapped present under the tree at Christmas.

"Chocolate chips!" I exclaimed.

On the cutting board I gave the chocolate a rough chop. Then, I eyed the unopened box of essential oils in the kitchen pantry. I pulled out a vial with the words "peppermint" on it. I let the vanilla bean gelato in the freezer sit on the counter until it was soft. I scooped about two cups out into a bowl, stirred in one drop of the mint oil into it, then folded in the chunks of chocolate. Sitting on the deck with my DIY peppermint chocolate gelato, I studied my wasteland. Blame the burst of mental energy on the peppermint oil. It was like I transcended to a town in Italy instead of being in the Sierras of California. As the music concert sounds bellowed and fireworks boomed, I was calm—I didn't care. I give credit to the peppermint oil.

Cooking with Essential Oils

When I wrote a few articles and a small booklet on essential oils twenty years ago, I did not include any food recipes infused with edible essential oils. Yes, people did use culinary oils then and before, but for the mainstream audience and essential oil companies, it wasn't popular. But times are a changing.

Two decades later, I've noticed culinary oils in the kitchen are a trend that continues to blossom. But it seems like edible recipes are far and few and sandwiched somewhere in some aromatherapy and essential oils books. I'm here to help! But note you have to know *exactly* how to include these oils, and which ones are edible, before you just dive into cooking and baking.

Ummm! What Smells So Good?

It's time to get cooking! You want to use food-grade edible essential oils, also called dietary or culinary essential oils. You want them to be from well-known brands, such as LorAnn Oils (which I use) or doTerra. Make sure they are not fragrance oils. And absolutely do not use medicinal oils, such as eucalyptus and tea tree essential oils stored in your bathroom cabinet. Like olive oil, it's good to know and trust your source for peace of mind and safety's sake to keep out added solvents, extenders, alcohol, or other fillers. Also, the U.S. Food & Drug

Administration offers an online published list of essential oils (solvent-free) that are "generally recognized as safe" (GRAS) to consume in beverages and foods.[1]

Next, remember the "toothpick" method of incorporating an essential oil into food. It gives you more control than using drops. When I had to give my cat a liquid medication, I used a dropper that had mL markings on it, which made it easier for me to know I was using the correct amount.

The thing is, glass eye droppers used for essential oils are not always calibrated. Yes, the majority of essential oil vials do have dropper inserts that help you control getting drops to drip one at a time. However, the holes vary in size and oil consistency differs, so it's not a precise measurement of a drop. That said, when using oils for cooking, the toothpick method is best done by dipping a toothpick into the essential oil; this is the best way to monitor using a small amount of oil (it can be a droplet) in food.

Also, it's best to dilute the essential oils just like you do for therapeutic, beauty, and cleaning recipes. I recommend for most food recipes to pair your essential oil with olive oil, part of the Mediterranean Diet. Other liquids you can use to dilute edible essential oils include vegetable oils, water, juice, and honey.

When I asked essential oils guru Kurt Schnaubelt of the Pacific Institute of Aromatherapy about using oils in cooking, he dished out his words of wisdom. "There have been repeated efforts to make culinary use of oils a popular science, but somehow these efforts fell a little short. A likely reason is that finding the proper dilution of essential oils becomes the challenge," he says. "This is overcome by some products where the oils are already appropriately diluted."

Cooking with essential oils is controversial among essential oil proponents. However, some top aromatherapists do encourage using raw essential oils for cooking and baking. It is advised to dilute food-grade essential oils with carrier oils such as olive oil or coconut oil in savory cuisine; maple syrup or honey for sweet fare to disperse the essential oil well.

When cooking with heat, it is recommended to add essential oils last to a recipe. This way, you'll preserve the flavor of the oil and it will not be over processed—helping to reap some of its antioxidants.

Why Cook with Essential Oils, Anyhow?

Cost and convenience are part of the package when you cook and bake with essential oils. I love using fresh food. No canned stuff for me, right? Well, unless you live on a farm that produces herbs like lavender or basil, you may be in for a rude awakening. The cost of fresh herbs can be high. One package of lavender can run you up to ten dollars. Also, you have to use it quickly or it will expire, whereas the shelf life of a vial of lavender essential oil is at least twofold and you'll only be using one or two drops.

When cooking a dish, I often get creative and want to add an exotic flair to it. Essential oils come to the rescue, again. Let's pretend I'm making a no bake lime mousse dessert for a hot summer day, and the key limes I purchased are less than what I expected—not especially juicy or sweet. I add a drop of lime essential oil and the light green mousse in ramekins topped with homemade whipped cream and key lime rind work for both texture and taste. Speaking of flavor . . .

Essential oils not only enhance aroma but zest! What happens if you do take a trek to get lavender and bring it home to infuse it in a baked good? It may not be as aromatic and flavorful as your trusty essential oil. After all the work you put into making a lavender-infused creation, if it's bland, it will be disappointing.

Not to forget using a few drops from a glass bottle is easy and convenient, whereas if you use the lavender herb, you'll have to grind it, wash the grinder and the cutting board. But there's more . . .

We know essential oils contain antioxidants and when paired with antioxidant-rich foods, including fruits and vegetables, you get a double punch of goodness. True, nutritionists and scientists do not know exactly how much we're getting, similar to consuming red wine vinegar, which contains resveratrol—but it's there! And yes, I'd rather have the "life blood" of plants in my recipes and food on the table instead of artificial flavorings, wouldn't you?

Essential Oils for Cooking and Baking

A variety of food-grade essential oils can be edible. However, it's essential for you to know that less is more, because the taste can be very potent.

Essential Oil	Flavor	Uses
Basil	Nutty, strong	Dips, pesto, pastas, salads, soups, sauces, tomatoes
Chamomile, Roman	Sweet, mild	Cakes, cookies, tea
Cinnamon	Spicy, warm	Cakes, cookies, scones
Geranium	Floral	Frosting, salads
Ginger	Sweet and savory	Cakes, cookies, scones, sauces
Lemon	Tart, sweet, light	Cakes, chicken, fish, muffins, salads
Orange	Sweet, light	Breads, chicken, muffins
Peppermint	Minty	Candy, cookies, cakes, tea
Rosemary	Strong, pungent	Breads, poultry, salads, scones, sauces, soups
Spearmint	Minty	Ice cream, sauces, tea

Some other food-grade essential oils are anise, bergamot, blood orange, clove, lemongrass, lime, nutmeg, oregano, tangerine, thyme, and wintergreen.

There are four groups of essential oils used in cooking, including citrus, floral, herbs, and spices. Now let me share how these can enhance dishes and turn them into a gastronomic delight:

Citrus Essential Oils: These edible oils, including blood orange, lemon, lime, and tangerine, work well with salad dressings drizzled over fruit and/or greens or desserts, such as chocolate cakes paired with blueberries and strawberries, and vegetables, including kale and spinach. Also, they can flavor up fish from salmon to shrimp and poultry like chicken or turkey.

Herb Essential Oils: These edible oils include rosemary, basil, and thyme. They work well used in savory breads and muffins, such as corn or pumpkin. They also can be beneficial in fish and poultry casseroles and vegetable or fish soups.

Floral Essential Oils: These edible oils do a good job making vanilla frostings, gelato, and ice cream, such as geranium or rose to cold drinks.

Spice Essential Oils: These edible oils include cinnamon, nutmeg, and cardamom. They are superb for sauces if you like some heat, such as tomato sauce, or baked pies like pumpkin or sweet potato and sweet and savory cakes, especially during colder months, and beverages. Indeed spicy culinary essential oils provide heat and flavor any time of year.

SEASONAL ESSENTIAL OILS AND FOUR SEASONS

Most of the essential oils I share in this section are from my top 20 picks, but I do include some other ones because they fit the season and complement one another.

WINTER

It's the Season: Shorter days, longer nights and often chilly temperatures call for hot, comfort food. During the holiday season, festive food, like hearty casseroles, soups, muffins, breads, puddings, and pies are commonplace. Then, when the New Year arrives it's not uncommon to want to eat clean food and get a fresh start. Immune-enhancing, mood-boosting, warming aromas are scents that come with wintertime. They can be found in plant-based salads, vegetarian casseroles, and soups, with lighter desserts.

Healing Winter Recipes: Biscotti, breads, casseroles, cakes and scones are popular foods to warm you up, and essential oils can give recipes extra flavor, especially when seasonal citrus or herbs are not available.

Winter Culinary Essential Oils: Anise, clove, cinnamon, ginger, nutmeg, and peppermint.

SPRING

It's the Season: As the days are longer, the weather is warmer, spring fever hits home. During the springtime it's commonplace to get a burst of energy as well as want to eat less, move more. And that's when our diet changes along with fresh fruits and vegetables. Energizing, floral, and herbaceous are the scents that welcome a renewal of a season after winter.

Healing Spring Recipes: Fresh fruits and vegetables, herbal teas, salads, and pasta plates are lighter fare than winter cuisine. These foods, many water-dense, can help you rejuvenate, energize, and detox your body.

Spring Culinary Essential Oils: Geranium, jasmine, lavender, lemon, orange, and rose.

SUMMER

It's the Season: Longer days, warmer nights call for a change in meals. Lighter meals, outdoor eating to fit the celebration of fun and sun. Cooling, energizing, floral, light fragrances are part of summertime.

Healing Summer Recipes: An array of fresh fruits and vegetables entice us to eat more of a plant-based diet. That means more salads, cheese plates, continental breakfasts or brunches, and fresh fish on the grill.

Summer Culinary Essential Oils: Chamomile, lemon, lavender, orange, sage, and spearmint.

FALL

It's the Season: Autumn is a time of change and the foliage is a reminder, with leaves changing color, the sun is setting earlier, and fall cleanup and nesting is all part of the time of year. Spicy, warming, woody scents blended with citrus notes are perfect for fall.

Healing Fall Recipes: Warm dishes like hot cereals, pancakes and waffles with maple syrup, hearty soups, vegetable casseroles, and fruit cobblers are part of the fall harvest.

Fall Culinary Essential Oils: Basil, cinnamon, ginger, lavender, nutmeg, and orange.

THE SEASONAL ESSENTIAL OILS
FOUR-DAY MENU PLAN

This four-day "Essential Oils Diet" is a sample menu including one day for each of the four seasons. The rest of the week or season is up to you. The menu is based on the Mediterranean Diet plan, which I have been following for decades.

When I used to write diet articles for women's magazines, I was often asked to create slim-down diets. One memory takes me back more than twenty years ago. I based the diets on California foods—it was the way I ate, fresh fruits, vegetables, whole grains, nuts, eggs, and some poultry. It was easy to create and was a spin-off of the diet plans I wrote with nutritionists, but instead of their picks, I chose fresh fare without counting calories and fat. It was fun and real.

But now, even though my eating style is still similar, it's a bit more sophisticated. Enter essential culinary oils. I'm infusing fresh food recipes with essential oils—remember, a toothpick method (small amount) is recommended because of the potency of the oils. Each day and each recipe includes foods found in the Mediterranean pyramid and foods chart.

And many of the essential oils—and olive oil, which is part of the Oldways Diet—will help you slim down, stay slim, and healthy up. So, let me take you out of your comfort zone and get ready to smell and taste the foods infused with essential oils.

Recipes (marked withy an asterish, *) can be found at the end of previous chapters (I suggest dog-ear the ones you want to try), or in the last chapter full of recipes. Go ahead—switch the days or seasons to fit you and your lifestyle. It is a basic menu plan to show you how to incorporate edible oils into your eating style.

Autumn is my number-one season. . . .

Day 1 FALL

Breakfast:
Cinnamon Rolls*
1 glass of orange juice, freshly squeezed or fortified brand
¾ cup whole grain cereal, ½ cup sliced banana, with ½ cup low-fat
  organic milk

Lunch:
Rice Salad with Ginger Oil Dressing*
1 cup cruciferous vegetables

Snack:
1 apple
1 cup hot chocolate

Dinner:
Rosemary, Thyme, Parsley Spaghetti*
Snack
½ cup vanilla bean gelato mixed with toothpick drop cinnamon
  essential oil

Day 2 WINTER

Breakfast:
Lemon Oil Raspberry Muffin*
1 cup fresh fruit, melon chunks
1 vegetarian omelet

Lunch:
California Clam Chowder*
Cornbread Thyme Muffin*

Snack:
Apple slices spread with peanut butter
1 (12-ounce) cup herbal tea

Dinner:
Roast Chicken with Rosemary*

1 cup kale mix with tomatoes drizzled with olive oil and red wine
  vinegar
1 baked potato, sweet or Russet, with pat of European-style butter

Snack:
Gingerbread Squares with Lemon Oil Frosting*

Day 3 SPRING

Breakfast:
1 cup hot water flavored with 1 drop lemon oil
Garden Fresh Smoothie*

Lunch:
Tuna Salad Italian Baguette*
1 cup fresh berries

Snack:
1 cup iced tea
Coconut Geranium Cookie*

Dinner:
Grilled Salmon in Spinach Leaves and Grape Compote*

Snack:
Orange Crème Brûlée*

Day 4 SUMMER

Breakfast:
¾ cup Greek yogurt
½ cup fresh fruit
1 bagel with cream cheese

Lunch:
Egg Rolls with Crab Filling
  and Lemon Fish Sauce*

Snack:
California Citrus Salsa Dip and Chips*

Dinner:
Grilled chicken
Sage Cheese Cornbread*

Snack:
Fresh fruit
Herbal tea

Okay, are you ready for the aromatic menu? I'm dishing up a variety of recipe categories to show you how cooking with essential oils can feed your senses and change it up in the kitchen. Enjoy yourself and have fun creating flavorful recipes with culinary oils that smell wonderful all year long.

Imagine you're baking a fresh apple pie in the fall. Oops! You forgot to replenish your supply of ground cinnamon. What do you do? Cinnamon essential oil comes to the rescue! Or what if you're making a savory pasta dish and want to include basil? It's too expensive fresh and you want your Mediterranean recipe to be extra flavorful—basil oil will do the trick. Essential oils can always be available in your pantry like a constant friend.

SCENT-SATIONAL HEALING OILS SHORT & SWEET

✓ Be aware adding essential oils to your diet can be a convenient, flavorful, and a healthful experience.
✓ Remember if you overheat essential oils while cooking, you'll lose their healing antioxidants . . .
✓ And note, storing essential oils in a cool, dry place will preserve the flavor and potency of their healing compounds.
✓ Caution: Vegetable carrier oils like olive oil can go rancid after their expiration dates have passed. Be sure to note the date and replace as needed.
✓ Be savvy and use specific essential oils to save money and enjoy extra flavor in dishes to celebrate Mother Nature's four seasons— and enjoy the warming and cooling benefits to match the time of year.

Edible Essentials Menu

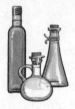

Much virtue in Herbs, little in Men.
—BENJAMIN FRANKLIN, Poor Richard's Almanac

One late Christmas afternoon after walking the dog, my brother told me that the lavender scones in the oven smelled good and looked picture-perfect. The floral aroma filled the air as the pastry cooled. I drizzled each triangle with an orange oil glaze. When I served one to my sibling, his blue eyes met mine.

After taking two bites, he said, "They're impeccable."

It was an aha moment because it linked to what I imagined my mom would say in a make-believe lavender farm kitchen at the beginning of this book. I felt a connectedness to family, which happens when scents and memories take you to places in the heart.

It was the familiar aromas of cinnamon, lavender, pine, and vanilla that triggered fond remembrances, the kind that make you feel good. Familiar flavors and scents give the eternal gift of family and home.

EDIBLE ESSENTIALS MENU

Bars, Muffins, Scones, Smoothies

While fresh foods are ideal, essential oils can add flavor to many dishes cooked up for breakfast. A serving of eggs can be enhanced with a culinary essential oil, such as basil. Baked goods in the morning are even tastier with citrusy essential oils, like orange. Not to leave out fragrant and spicy oils like cinnamon. And fresh fruit with a hint of a floral essential oil like lavender can be heavenly. Seasonal berries can be drizzled with a drop of lemon oil for a fresh effect (especially if you don't have lemons on hand) and then paired with hot chocolate and a hint of peppermint for a breakfast feast.

Ginger Granola Bars
Lavender Scones with Orange Glaze
Lemon Oil Raspberry Muffins
Pumpkin Spice Bars with Sage Oil Frosting

Ginger Granola Bars

Granola bars are a must-have breakfast snack year-round. These bars, which are a mix of nature's fall foods, include dried fruit, honey, nuts, oats, and seeds, molded into a rectangular bar. These easy to make bars are convenient, and taste crazy good, especially if they're homemade. Granola bars take me back to the seventies. I made crunchy granola in friends' kitchenettes so I could take them on the road with me, always fantasizing about having my own kitchen. Today boxes of granola bars at your grocery store are okay, but making your own and adding essential oils for extra flavor and aroma are worth the time and effort.

2 cups old-fashioned rolled oats
½ cup walnuts, rough chop
½ cup brown sugar
3 tablespoons European-style butter
¾ cup honey
¼ cup molasses
1 teaspoon pure vanilla extract
1 drop cinnamon essential oil
1 drop ginger essential oil
½ cup dried crystalized ginger, chopped
European-style butter, melted (a bit for greasing
    baking dish)

In a pan place the oats and nuts. Bake at 350 degrees F for about 10 minutes. Remove. Set aside. In a saucepan, combine sugar, butter, honey, and molasses. On medium heat, stir and heat until mixture boils, remove. Add extract and oils. Stir. Fold in oats, nuts, and dried ginger. Butter a square baking dish. Bake at 300 degrees F for about 15 to 20 minutes. Note: For chewier bars, bake less than more. Remove from oven and cool. Cut into bars. Store in airtight contain in refrigerator.

Makes 10 to 12 bars.

Your kitchen will smell heavenly like a cookie shop. You'll love munching on the granola bar with your name on it. You can add any ingredients, including chocolate chips, coconut, dried berries—and other spice essential oils, such as nutmeg or citrusy oils like lemon or orange. If you want to get fancy, melt white or dark chocolate chips in the microwave (about 30 seconds, stir until melted). Drizzle on top or dip bar bottom. Either way works and you'll enjoy your personalized granola bars for all seasons.

Lavender Scones with Orange Glaze

❖ ❖ ❖

Drop scones, triangle scones, mini scones, a circle scone—they're all dear to me. One afternoon when I was sitting on the deck, an acquaintance stopped by. She told me that she liked my scone recipes in the town newspaper. She added that frosting, globs of it, made them more flavorful, and so tasty that she revised my recipe and sold the scones. Speechless, I took the high road . . . but I did change up one of my scone recipes and yes, it is palatable with a European flair of lavender and orange essential oils.

2 cups cake flour
½ cup all-purpose flour
1 tablespoon baking powder
¼ cup granulated sugar
5 tablespoons European-style butter, chilled cubes
1 organic egg
⅔ cup organic buttermilk
*1 teaspoon lavender leaves (provides a pleasing look
    and texture)*
1 teaspoon vanilla extract
1 drop lavender essential oil
½ cup almonds, chopped fine

In a bowl, combine flours, baking powder, and sugar. Add butter. Set aside. In another bowl, combine egg, buttermilk, lavender leaves, vanilla extract, and lavender oil. Fold in almonds. On a parchment-lined baking sheet, place drops of batter (use a ⅓ cup ice cream scoop). Bake at 350 degrees F for about 20 minutes or until golden brown. Cool.

Serves 12.

ORANGE GLAZE

1 cup confectioners sugar
¼ cup half-and-half
1 teaspoon lemon rind
1 teaspoon vanilla extract
1 drop maple syrup
1 drop orange essential oil

In a small bowl, combine sugar, half-and-half, lemon rind, and vanilla. Mix in syrup and orange oil. Blend with a mixer until smooth. Drizzle lightly on scones.

Lemon Oil Raspberry Muffins

On a trip to Monterey-Pacific Grove in the early spring I had fantasized before leaving that I'd enjoy an appetizing breakfast with a view of the sea. Well, it didn't happen like that exactly. I ended up munching on a vending machine fruit muffin. I finished savoring my coffee and vowed to make a fresh tasty citrusy muffin from scratch to write home about.

1 lemon (cut in half and use juice)
½ cup organic 2 percent low-fat milk
½ cup European style butter (soft or melted)
¼ cup granulated white sugar
2 organic eggs
2 cups cake flour
1 tablespoon baking powder
1 drop lemon essential oil
1 teaspoon olive oil
½ to ¾ cup fresh raspberries, lightly rinsed with water, sliced in half
Extra fresh raspberries, whole (for garnish)

1 cup confectioners sugar
3 tablespoons fresh lemon juice
1 drop lemon essential oil (use a toothpick for a tiny
    drop)
1 teaspoon honey

Combine all ingredients and stir until smooth. Use immediately or put into refrigerator until ready to use.

In a large bowl, stir together juice and milk. Set aside. Cream butter and sugar. Add eggs, flour, and baking powder. Mix well. Add juice and milk. Stir in lemon oil and olive oil. Fold in raspberries. Fill muffin cups in tin pan with batter. (Use a ½ cup ice cream scoop to make muffins the same size.) Bake 20 minutes or until tops are light golden brown and firm to touch. Cool and remove from pan. Drizzle with glaze. Remove muffin wrappers for a nicer look. Top with a few raspberries. Breakfast muffins store well in an airtight container.

Makes about 8.

This recipe is easy to make. The fresh flavor provides notes of tart citrus and bursts of sweet berries. The decadent glaze is a nice touch so a small amount is best. The flour offers a light, fluffy volume and butter is better than vegetable oil for taste. These fruity muffins are unforgettable paired with fresh squeezed orange juice and super coffee (I ordered Douse Egberts ground coffee online).

Pumpkin Spice Bars with Sage Oil Frosting

❖ ❖ ❖

Autumn is my much-loved season, a time for aromatic pumpkin and spice. I decided to add an herbal touch to this recipe inspired by my friend's old-fashioned pumpkin bars. My goal was to marry sweet and savory flavors and scents. It reminded me of a trip to a pumpkin patch with the spectacular oranges and reds and yellows of the season lining the roads. Not only are the colors fall-ish, the taste and smell are perfect during a colder season when we turn to foods with a warming taste for comfort.

Oil for greasing roll pan
4 eggs
2 cups sugar [Author's note: You can cut the amount in
    half if preferred.]
⅓ cup Marsala Olive Oil
1 (16-ounce) can pumpkin
2 cups flour
1 teaspoon baking powder
2 teaspoons cinnamon
½ teaspoon ginger
¼ teaspoon cloves
½ cup raisin or currants
½ cup pecans or walnuts, chopped ginger

Heat oven to 350 degrees F. Grease jelly roll pan, 15½ by 1½ by 2 inches. Beat eggs, sugar, olive oil, and pumpkin in mixing bowl. Stir in dry ingredients. Mix in raisins and nuts. Pour batter into prepared pan. Bake until golden brown, about 25 to 30 minutes, cool. Frost as desired, cut into bars, about 2 inches by 1½ inches.

Makes 49.

(Courtesy: *Cooking with California Olive Oil: Treasured Family Recipes*, by Gemma Sanita Sciabica)

SAGE FROSTING

*1 cup confectioners sugar (add more if you prefer a
    thicker consistency)*
6 ounces cream cheese, softened or whipped variety
1 teaspoon vanilla extract
1 drop sage essential oil
1 teaspoon maple syrup
Pumpkin seeds, shelled

In a small bowl blend sugar and cream cheese. Add vanilla. Mix in sage oil and maple syrup. Blend until creamy. Frost bars. Top with seeds.

ESSENTIAL OILS-INFUSED ASSORTED APPETIZERS

California Citrus Oil Salsa and Chips
Egg Rolls with Crab Filling and Lemon Oil Fish Sauce

California Citrus Oil Salsa and Chips

After the spring trip to Monterey, I cherished the images of colorful fruits and vegetables at the roadside produce stands of Moss Landing. The tomatoes not only inspired me to make a fresh tomato garlic sauce for pasta, but they also urged me to make fresh salsa spiked with essential oils for a more California flavor. This recipe is inspired by my love for fresh tomatoes—not canned—and a variety of citrus notes.

4 fresh large Roma or vine tomatoes, diced
4 tablespoons red onion or scallions, diced
2 small chili peppers, diced
1 teaspoon cilantro
2 teaspoons fresh lime juice
1 drop lemon essential oil
1 teaspoon extra virgin olive oil
Ground pepper and sea salt to taste
Parmesan cheese shavings

In a mixing bowl, add tomatoes and onion, mix well. Fold in peppers, cilantro, and citrus juice. Mix in essential oil and olive oil. Add spices. Place in refrigerator for at least 30 minutes. When ready to serve, top with cheese.

Serves 3 or 4.

Semi-Homemade Chips

Canola oil to grease skillet
3–4 flour tortillas
1 drop basil essential oil
1 drop lime essential oil
¼ cup olive oil

In a skillet, cover the bottom about ¼ inch with canola oil. Set aside. Cut round tortillas into triangles like a pizza pie. Once the oil sizzles on medium heat, place tortilla triangles into the pan. Turn a few times until the chips are light brown on both sides. Remove. Place on paper towels to absorb oil. Mix basil and lime essential oils with olive oil. Drizzle on top of chips. Toss chips to mix in oils. Serve warm with salsa.

Serves 3 or 4.

Egg Rolls with Crab Filling and Lemon Fish Sauce

Egg rolls are a treat with Chinese takeout or solo. I went through an egg roll phase. At the grocery store deli, they offer hot ready-to-eat egg rolls. Each shopping visit, I'd order a few but once at the checkout line, the small bag of rolls was empty. I'd blush and pay. That's when I decided to find a failproof recipe and make my own Asian treats to serve with vegetables and rice.

12 egg roll wrappers (7 inches by 7 inches)
Crab filling
Marsala olive oil for brushing rolls

Place 1 egg wrapper on working surface, with 1 corner toward you. Spoon about ¼ cup filling in center. Place corner under filling. Fold left and right corners over filling, overlapping at center. Brush last corner with water, roll egg roll away from you, onto the moistened corner. Brush rolls on all sides with olive oil. Place on a foil-lined greased baking sheet. Bake at 325 degrees F for 10 to 15 minutes or until golden. Serve with sauce of your choice.

Makes 12.

CRAB FILLING

½ pound crab (picked over), cooked
¾ pound sole, salmon fillets or shrimp, cooked (choose one)
¾ cup water chestnuts, chopped
2 green onions, finely chopped
2 tablespoons catchup
1 tablespoon soy sauce
1 tablespoon lime or lemon juice
1 egg
2 garlic cloves, minced

Chop crab and sole until minced, place in mixing bowl. Add chestnuts, onions, catchup, soy sauce, lime juice, egg, and garlic. Use about ¼ cup filling for each egg roll.

(Courtesy: *Cooking with California Olive Oil: Treasured Family Recipes* by Gemma Sanita Sciabica)

LEMON FISH SAUCE

½ cup peanuts, ground
1 small chili, minced
2 tablespoons honey
2 tablespoons lime juice
2 garlic cloves, minced
¾ cup cilantro, chopped
1/3 cup light olive oil
1 drop ginger essential oil
1 drop lemon essential oil

In a small bowl, combine nuts, chili, honey, lime juice, garlic, and cilantro. Combine olive oil, ginger, and lemon oils. Drizzle over egg rolls. Note: You can steam white or brown rice, and add a mix of cruciferous vegetables. Now you can have delicious and healthful takeout right at home!

ESSENTIAL OILS–INFUSED SALADS

Salads are my preferred food—and now essential oils also play a role. Kale and cabbage mixed with lemon oil, baby spinach and feta cheese drizzled with a basil oil dressing, and pasta with crucifers tossed with a taste of orange oil. It's all delicious. Adding dressings infused with essential oils work for a burst of flavors. Not only do they add notes of deliciousness to a salad, adding herbal and citrusy notes, but they can provide a taste that might not be currently available. If you don't have fresh lemons or garden basil, essential oils are a substitute to give a dressing that special kick.

Fruit Salad with Lavender Oil Dressing
Rice Salad with Ginger Oil Dressing

Fruit Salad with Lavender Oil Dressing

In college I lived on fruit salad and bagels. The Student Union bagel bar was heaven to me. One evening before my last class I stared at the wall menu of bagel combos. I chose the number with cream cheese, tomatoes, and a poppy seed bagel. A fruit salad accompanied the bagel. It was basic—apples, grapes, oranges, and melon chunks. I was content eating and studying before my geology class. This recipe from Gemma Sciabica is full of California goodness with its fruit, avocado, and nuts paired with my earthy lavender oil dressing. I know it will rock your world like it does mine.

4 apricots, sliced
1 cup pimiento stuffed olives, sliced

1 tablespoon poppy seeds
1 avocado, diced
2 peaches or nectarines in bite-size pieces
½ pound sweet cherries, pitted
1 cup dates, chopped
1 cup mozzarella or Swiss cheese, cubed
¼ cup pecans, pistachios, or pine nuts
½ cup cantaloupe or honeydew, balls or cubed
4 plums, sliced
1 cup blueberries or berries of your choice
1 cup pineapple tidbits
1 apple or pear diced (or grapes seedless)
4 fresh or dried figs, sliced
6 or 8 radicchio, red leaf, or Boston lettuce leaves

Combine all salad ingredients, spoon dressing on, toss gently. Line large shallow salad bowl with lettuce leaves. Arrange ingredients over lettuce. Garnish with sprigs of rose-scented geranium, unsprayed.

Serves 6.

(Courtesy: *Cooking with California Olive Oil: Treasured Family Recipes* by Gemma Sanita Sciabica)

Dressing

½ cup fresh orange juice
¼ cup honey
1 teaspoon pure vanilla extract
⅓ cup olive oil
1 drop lemon essential oil
½ drop lavender essential oil

Combine all ingredients in a blender. Mix well.

Serves 6.

Rice Salad with Ginger Oil Dressing

❖ ❖ ❖

Rice salads are different—they're not your run-of-the-mill green salad with tomatoes, right? I found this flavorful rice salad complete with chicken, vegetables, rice, and paired it with a ginger oil dressing that I created. It's a mix of twentieth- and twenty-first-century cooking, and its combination of sweet and spicy notes has an extra wow factor.

½ pound chicken baked or grilled, chopped
1 avocado, diced
2 cups rice, long grain, cooked
⅓ cup fresh basil, parsley, or cilantro, chopped
1 medium cucumber, diced
4 yellow or red tomatoes, chopped
1 cup corn kernels or green beans, cooked
1 red, yellow, or green bell pepper, minced
1 cup fresh mushrooms, sliced, sautéed in a little
    olive oil
1 cup peas or dried beans, cooked
1 cup water chestnuts, sliced
2 cups strawberries or berries of your choice
1 orange or tangerine segments
4 cups mixed baby lettuce or spinach

In a large bowl, mix all salad ingredients, chicken, avocado, rice, basil, parsley, cucumber, tomatoes, corn, bell pepper, mushrooms, peas, water chestnuts, berries, and citrus. Line a large shallow serving bowl or platter with lettuce. In a bowl whisk together dressing ingredients (recipe below). Pour over salad, toss gently. Spoon onto lettuce-lined plate.

Serves 4.

(Courtesy: *Cooking with California Olive Oil* by Gemma Sanita Sciabica)

GINGER OIL DRESSING

⅓ cup olive oil
¼ cup fresh lemon juice
1–2 tablespoons soy sauce
Sea salt and ground black pepper to taste
½ drop ginger essential oil
½ drop orange essential oil
¼ cup sesame seeds

In a bowl combine oil, lemon juice, soy sauce, salt and pepper. Add ginger and orange oils. Fold in seeds.

Serves 4.

MEDITERRANEAN SANDWICHES

Tacos with Greek Guacamole and Lime Oil
Tuna Lemon Salad Italian Baguette
Turkey and Spinach Wraps Italian-Style

Sandwiches can be a quick food to eat or a delicious food to remember. So instead of making an ordinary fast-food taco, homemade tuna sandwich on basic bread, or a store-bought wrap, it's time to get your essential oil on and enjoy fab flavors! Mediterranean sandwiches, like these, provide TLC and you'll feel like you're in a European café munching on a culinary delight thanks to these edible essential oils.

Tacos with Greek Guacamole and Lime Oil

I often order vegetarian tacos. One time my male companion was embarrassed to place my order to the man in the drive-thru window:

He mumbled, "Please leave out the beans and meat."

My carnivore mate clearly felt I was making him look silly. I get it. Meatless tacos were odd. This recipe is a compromise, using poultry with a tart lime essential oil in the guacamole mixture (below the taco recipe) for a twist.

¼ cup Marsala Olive Fruit Oil
1 onion, sliced
1 bell pepper, diced
½ pound lean turkey
½ cup cabbage head, chopped or shredded (about
   ½ pound)

1 cup fresh mushrooms, chopped
2 chilies, chopped
1 cup cilantro, chopped
¼ cup hot taco sauce
4 taco shells
1 cup cheddar cheese, shredded
½ cup olives, sliced

In a large skillet, add oil, onion, pepper, and turkey. Cook over medium heat until well browned. Add cabbage, lower heat, cover, cook about 10 minutes. Add mushrooms, chilies, cilantro, and hot sauce. Heat taco shells as label directs. Spoon turkey mixture into taco shells, cover with cheese and olives. Add a dollop of guacamole.

Serves 4.

(Courtesy: *Cooking with California Olive Oil: Popular Recipes* by Gemma Sanita Sciabica)

GREEK GUACAMOLE WITH LIME OIL

3 avocados, peeled and pitted
¼ cup Roma tomatoes
¼ cup red onion, chopped
2 tablespoons feta cheese
¼ cup black olives
2 tablespoons hot taco sauce
1 drop lime essential oil
Ground pepper and sea salt to taste

In a bowl, combine avocados, tomatoes, onion, cheese, and olives. Mix sauce and oil, stir into chunky mixture. Sprinkle with pepper and salt. Chill in fridge until ready to serve in tacos.

Serves 4.

Tuna Lemon Salad Italian Baguette

❖ ❖ ❖

Tuna salad is a twentieth-century favorite. In college I frequented the Bagel Bar. I recall ordering a tuna delight but it was not so delightful. No super mayo, herbs, onions, celery—just cat food–like canned fish on a plain bagel. This classic sandwich is an updated version of a food that can be flavorful with the right finesse. I concocted a tuna lemon baguette with albacore chunks of tuna, organic greens, tomatoes, herbs, spices, cheese, and an essential oil for an extra citrus kick.

1 (3-ounce) can of tuna, albacore packed in water
3 tablespoons store-bought mayonnaise infused with
    olive oil
1 drop lemon essential oil
2 teaspoons red onion, chopped
2 tablespoons fresh Mediterranean herbs, chopped
1 fresh artisan baguette (whole grain is preferred)
½ to 1 cup kale and spinach salad mix
½ cup Roma tomatoes, sliced
1 slice of Monterey Jack cheese

In a bowl, mix tuna with mayonnaise, lemon oil, onion, and herbs. Keep it chunky. Chill in refrigerator for at least one hour. When ready to make your new, improved tuna delight, cut a baguette in half. Spread with lettuce, tomatoes, and tuna. Top with a slice of cheese. Serves two open face sandwiches.

Or you can slice the baguette in diagonal slices to make more than less. Simply double the recipe if you have more family, friends, or neighbors to feed. Truth be told, this twist on tuna served on a baguette may surprise you with its burst of flavors, including the lemon oil. Not only are you getting lean protein, vegetables, and grains—you'll get plenty of taste without the sweat of cooking a meal.

Turkey and Spinach Wraps Italian-Style

❖ ❖ ❖

Wraps from food trucks and cafés can be filled with a load of calories and fat. If you make them at home, you control the ingredients. That means you can have your wrap and eat it, too, without gaining unwanted pounds, as long as you use, spices, herbs, condiments, and essential oils.

¼ *cup store-bought mayonnaise infused with olive oil*
1 drop basil or rosemary essential oil
2 tablespoons red wine vinegar
Dash of ground black pepper and sea salt
4 (8-inch) whole grain flour tortillas
1 cup fresh spinach, chopped
⅓ *pound deli organic roasted turkey breast*
1 cup Swiss or Monterey Jack cheese, shredded/
4 tomato slices

In a bowl, combine mayonnaise, essential oil, vinegar, and spices. Spread half of mixture on top of each tortilla. Top with spinach and turkey. Spread turkey and spinach with rest of vinegar oil mixture. Top with tomatoes and cheese. Fold tortilla. Warm up in microwave or serve cold.

Serves 4.

SOUPS AND BREADS

California Clam Chowder with Herb Oil French Bread
Chicken Vegetable Soup with Thyme Cornbread Muffins
Lentil Soup with Lemon Oil Breadsticks
Potato Soup with Rosemary Crouton

Growing up in the fifties and sixties, boring soup was a staple for my family. It was often served on those busy school and work nights or for lunch on the weekends. Canned soups, including tomato and pea, were my foes, whereas, turkey noodle and minestrone were okay. I love chunky homemade soup and bread—all types. Why? It's the fresh ingredients and essential oils that spice up these soups and breads that make them a memorable meal for me these days.

California Clam Chowder with Herb Oil French Bread

On a road trip, my friends wanted to stop at a popular Deep South spot known for its clam chowder. I was on a juice detox fast to drop five pounds so I passed. It was a soup and bread event I regret not experiencing. This is a California-style inspired clam chowder, with less sodium and fat. The tomato-based ingredients give it a Golden State–Mediterranean flavor complete with rosemary essential oil bread.

⅓ cup Marsala Olive Oil
2 slices Canadian bacon, lean, chopped
1 onion, small, chopped

1 cup celery, sliced
1 green chili, chopped (or ¼ habanero)
¼ cup flour
½ cup water
1 potato, chopped
1 cup basil, fresh, chopped
1 cup artichoke hearts, canned, drained, cut into
  bite-size pieces
1½ cups tomatoes, fresh or canned
1½ cups asparagus tips
1 avocado, diced
Salt to taste
2 (6½-ounce) cans clams, with liquid

In a Dutch oven add olive oil and bacon, cook 30 seconds. Add onion, celery and green chili. Cook stirring about 3 minutes. Stir in flour, water, potato, and basil. Cover, cook 10 minutes. Stir in artichoke hearts, tomatoes, asparagus, avocado, and salt, cook 2 minutes. Add clams, heat just below boiling point. Serve hot in tureen or individual bowls.

Serves 6.

(Courtesy: *Cooking with California Olive Oil: Recipes from the Heart for the Heart*, Gemma Sanita Sciabica)

HERB OIL FRENCH BREAD

3 tablespoons extra virgin olive oil
1 teaspoon European-style butter, melted
1 drop rosemary essential oil
1 teaspoon fresh thyme, chopped
Ground pepper to taste
1 loaf store-bought whole grain bread

In a small bowl whisk olive oil, butter, rosemary oil, thyme, pepper. Set aside. Slice bread. Spread tops with oil. Heat in oven until hot. Serve.

Chicken Vegetable Soup with Thyme Cornbread Muffins

Truth be told, I used to think soup was strictly canned and was only for when you got a cold or flu...or during a power outage. Once I mastered the art of making chunky, homemade soup, I changed my mind. Soup is tasty and essential oils give it extra flavor. Not only is it easy to do but the aroma in the kitchen and anticipation of the chunky goodness in a bowl is worth the wait. One non-traditional Thanksgiving, I served a chicken not the big turkey. The next day, I made chicken soup. I didn't have fresh basil for a Mediterranean flavor, so instead I used the basil essential oil that was sitting in my pantry. The end result? It was a flavorful soup to love!

So here's to soup lovers, but remember, less is more when tossing in salt and essential oils.

1 organic chicken (2 pounds)
¼ cup carrots, diced
½ cup celery, diced
½ cup onion, diced
¾ cup Roma tomatoes, diced
¼ cup extra virgin olive oil
1 drop basil essential oil
Sea salt and ground pepper to taste

In a large pot, put chicken inside, cover with water. Bring to a boil. Lower heat to a simmer. Cook chicken. Remove and put in bowl. Debone chicken, chop into chunks. Strain chicken broth and put it in another soup pan. Add carrots, celery, onion, and tomatoes. Cook on medium heat until vegetables are tender. Add chicken to broth and vegetables. Stir in olive oil, basil oil, salt, and pepper.

Serves 8.

Thyme Cornbread Muffins

For years I used the store-bought small box of cornbread mix because it was convenient and fail-proof. Then, one day I purchased a box of cornmeal and used it! The epiphany of making cornbread from scratch and adding fresh herbs or an herbal essential oil is the key to turning a boring square of cornbread into a culinary delight.

1¼ cups all-purpose flour
2 teaspoons baking powder
½ cup low-fat organic milk
½ cup low-fat organic buttermilk
¼ cup extra virgin olive oil
2 brown eggs

SPREAD

½ cup European-style butter
¼ cup honey
1 drop thyme essential oil

In a bowl, combine flour and baking powder. Add milk, buttermilk, oil, and eggs. Pour batter into paper-lined muffin tin. Bake at 400 degrees F for 15 to 20 minutes until light golden brown and firm to touch. Remove. Cool. Melt butter in a pan or microwave. Once melted, add honey and stir in essential oil. Spread mixture on top of muffins.

Makes 12.

Lentil Soup with Lemon Oil Breadsticks

Being a Mediterranean Diet devotee, it seems off that I don't like beans. Blame it on their fuzzy texture, which brings me back to second-grade lunch. Beans and I never made up. But I started to eat lentils, sparingly. If they're in a chunky vegetable homemade soup, like this recipe, with an herbal essential oil, I barely know they're there. Which is great because I'm getting the lentil nutrients, including fiber and protein, *and* they're low in fat and calories.

1 cup dry lentils
5 cups water
5 cups organic vegetarian broth
½ onion, chopped
3 cloves garlic, chopped
1 cup celery, diced
1 cup carrots, diced
3 cups tomatoes, fresh, chopped
1 cup pasta shells
¼ cup olive oil
¼ drop basil essential oil
Ground pepper and sea salt to taste

In a colander rinse lentils, put in a pot. Add water, broth, onion, garlic, celery, carrots, and tomatoes. Cook over low heat. Cover pot with lid for about a half hour or until lentils are tender. In a separate pan, cook pasta. Drain. Add to soup. Stir in olive oil and basil oil. Add pepper and salt.

Serves 10.

LEMON OIL BREADSTICKS

Place sticks onto a parchment-covered baking sheet. Warm in a 350-degree F oven. Remove and sprinkle with Parmesan cheese. In a microwave, melt ¼ cup European-style butter and ¼ drop essential lemon. Drizzle with mixture. Place in a napkin-lined bread basket.

Potato Soup with Rosemary Croutons

As a kid I liked two kinds of soup, sort of. Lipton's Chicken and Rice (in a box), and Campbell's Turkey Noodle were go-to choices. One weekend, my mom made a potato soup from scratch. I asked for my typical turkey or chicken broths. But I didn't win. I reluctantly dipped my spoon into the thick, creamy flavorful soup. After the first bite, my soup repertoire expanded. This recipe uses fresh basil, which can be substituted with flavorful and convenient basil essential oil, available year-round. Pair it with rosemary oil croutons for the aromatic taste that'll wow your palate.

¼ cup Marsala Olive Fruit Oil
3 large potatoes, diced
1 onion, chopped (or leeks)
6 garlic cloves, chopped or 1 head of garlic, roasted
1 bell pepper, diced
1 small cabbage, shredded
2 bay leaves
6 cups chicken or beef broth
Salt, pepper, cayenne to taste
¼ cup fresh basil or parsley, chopped
1 cup cheddar, Monterey Jack or Swiss cheese, shredded
1½ cups croutons [See recipe below]

In a large skillet over medium heat add oil, potatoes, onion, garlic, bell pepper, and cabbage. Cook covered until vegetables are almost tender, then add bay leaves. In large pot combine broth with vegetables, bring to boil, lower to simmer. Cover and cook 20 to 30 minutes. Stir in salt, pepper, cayenne, and basil. Remove bay leaves, sprinkle with cheese. Serve with croutons.

Serves 4 to 6.

(Courtesy: *Cooking with California Olive Oil: Treasured Family Recipes* by Gemma Sanita Sciabica)

ROSEMARY CROUTONS

1 cup Italian whole grain bread, cubed
2 tablespoons olive oil
1 tablespoon European-style butter, melted
1 teaspoon minced garlic
¼ drop rosemary essential oil
Ground pepper and sea salt to taste

Cut bread into ½-inch cubes. Place bread onto a baking sheet. Drizzle with olive oil, butter, garlic, rosemary oil. Bake at 375 degrees F for about 10 minutes or until golden brown. Sprinkle with pepper and salt.

PASTA PLATES

Pasta Salad with a Citrus Twist
Penne Pasta with Stir-Fry Vegetables

Pasta and I have a long history. It was one of my foods of choice in college, after grad school, and during the Great Recession. After all, whole grain pasta is inexpensive and paired with vegetables it can be a meal—for me. The thing is, it can lack in flavor if you don't use extras like essential oils. And that is what makes pasta plates a gourmet meal for one or more with an aroma that can lure a crowd.

Pasta Salad with a Citrus Twist

Welcome to a summertime chilled pasta with an Italian twist, complete with olive oil and lemon essential oil. When I lived in the San Francisco Bay Area, I used to buy the ready-made deli pasta salad. But once living in the mountains, I ended up making more and more of the pre-pared dishes I loved back home. I never knew how easy this pasta salad with a tang was to put together from scratch until one hot summer day in the Sierra, surrounded by wildfires and poor air quality, I decided to make a cold salad to chill.

2 cups rotini, cooked
1 cup broccoli and cauliflower florets, steamed or
*   boiled*
½ cup cherry or grape tomatoes
¼ cup black olives, sliced
¼ cup artichoke hearts, chopped

½ cup cheese, Monterey Jack
¼ cup walnuts, chopped
¼ cup Parmesan cheese, shavings

In a bowl, combine rotini, vegetables, olives, artichokes, cheese, and walnuts. Top with Parmesan cheese. Put in refrigerator.

VINAIGRETTE DRESSING

¾-part olive oil
¼-part red wine vinegar
1 drop lemon essential oil
1 drop basil essential oil

Mix and put in refrigerator. When ready to serve drizzle dressing on top of pasta mixture.

Makes 3 to 4 servings.

To make this salad friendlier you can set it up like a pasta bar much like a potato or salad bar. In small ramekins, put a variety of ingredients, including vegetables, cheeses, nuts—all chopped. Let your family or guests build their own pasta salad. The very best part of mixing it up allows everyone to have cool down and fill up on the foods they love. And this makes a noodle salad a crowd pleaser.

Penne Pasta with Stir-Fry Veggies

This stir-fry meal takes me back to a time when I was in grad school. I went on a cooking strike (again) while studying for oral exams during Indian summer in the San Francisco Bay Area. One night an ex-boyfriend paid me a visit. He used a new wok I had received for a birthday present. It was so easy to concoct a vegetable dish, and it was fast and fresh, a perfect quick meal to make when it's too hot to cook. Translation: You can get out of the kitchen fast and leave cooking and baking for autumn when the air is crisp. Or use this recipe for fall and switch to seasonal vegetables.

2 cups cooked whole grain penne pasta (or tri-color
    penne)
1 tablespoon extra-virgin olive oil
1 tablespoon European-style butter
2 tablespoons red onion, chopped
¼ cup green bell pepper, chopped
¼ cup fresh spinach, chopped
¼ cup zucchini, chopped or sliced
¼ cup Roma tomatoes, sliced
Fresh basil (garnish)
Ground pepper and sea salt to taste

DRESSING

4 tablespoons extra virgin olive oil
1 drop lemon essential oil

In a saucepan, cook pasta in boiling water until al dente. While pasta is cooking, heat olive oil and butter in large sauté pan or wok over high heat. Add onion, bell pepper, spinach, zucchini, and tomatoes. Stir-fry until all ingredients are hot, vegetables tender. Cook for no longer than 5 minutes. Drain pasta. In a large dish, place pasta and fold in vegetables. Top with basil and spices. Drizzle with dressing.

Serves 4.

If you want to add lean protein, try 8 ounces jumbo shrimp, cooked, rinsed. Add to the vegetable mix and stir-fry along with the colorful bunch. This quickie dish hits the spot for lunch or dinner. Add slices of herbal bread from your favorite local bakery. And don't forget iced or hot tea with fresh lemon slices.

ESSENTIAL ENTRÉES

*Grilled Salmon in Spinach Leaves
and Grape Compote
Roast Chicken with Rosemary
Tuna Noodle Casserole*

As a grazer for decades, eating a large entrée isn't my style. But these three main dish recipes can be cooked up and dished out in smaller portions—working as entrées more than one time. Also, because of the essential oils with Mediterranean flavors, you can spruce up a salmon, chicken, or tuna meal and create a special dinner for you know who—or simply you. Enjoy!

Grilled Salmon in Spinach Leaves and Grape Compote

For some reason, salmon and men with me don't go well together. One date ruined the over-baked fish with bottled sauce and no herbs, spices, or essential oils. Another blind date dumped personal woes on me so I didn't eat my grilled salmon; instead I gave it to my beloved cat. I stayed clear of salmon until one afternoon when I found a recipe. My protest against this seafood was over. This Mediterranean-inspired recipe gave the fatty fish a romantic flair paired with the fruit compote complete with citrus and spicy essential oils.

1 egg white lightly beaten
4 ¾-inch slices salmon
4 tablespoons bread crumbs
½ cup fresh basil or parsley, chopped

¼ cup Marsala Olive Fruit Oil
4 garlic cloves, chopped
1 teaspoon celery seeds
½ teaspoon sage
Salt, pepper, and cayenne to taste
4 large spinach leaves, stems removed
¼ cup lemon juice
4 tablespoons pine nuts

In a pie plate add egg white, coat salmon on both sides. In another pie plate, add crumbs, basil, olive oil, garlic, celery seeds, sage, salt, pepper, and cayenne. Press salmon in crumb mixture on both sides. Place each slice on a spinach leaf, fold over to cover fish. Place packages, folded side down, in a wire basket with a handle. Grill about 4 inches above hot coals for about 4 minutes on each side, or until fish flakes easily when tested with fork. Place on serving platter, unwrap, drizzle with lemon juice, sprinkle with pine nuts.

Serves 4.

(Courtesy: *Cooking with California Olive Oil: Treasured Family Recipes* by Gemma Sanita Sciabica)

GRAPE COMPOTE

2 cups grapes, seedless (red)
2 tablespoons brown sugar
1/4 cup orange juice
1 teaspoon honey or maple syrup
1 drop orange essential oil
1 drop cinnamon essential oil

In a frying pan combine grapes, sugar, and juice. Cook over medium heat for about 5 minutes. Add honey or syrup with orange and cinnamon essential oils. Simmer for a few minutes. Serve with salmon.

Roast Chicken with Rosemary

Chicken and I have a history. I've boiled it for a sick dog; ate KFC when in need of a quick bite; and have made it for homemade soup when fighting a bug. On weekends, my mom made meals with TLC, like Roast Chicken with Rosemary. She used rosemary ground with olive oil for a rub. This recipe is based on my memory of the flavorful poultry and took me out of the rut of eating barbecue or fried chicken. It's a recipe with a hint of sophistication.

1 cup flour
Sea salt and ground pepper to taste
6 chicken breasts, skinless
⅓ cup olive oil
2 garlic cloves, chopped fine
¼ cup fresh orange juice
1 tablespoon extra virgin olive oil
1 drop rosemary essential oil
Sprigs of rosemary
Fresh orange slices

In a bowl, mix flour, salt, and pepper. Dip chicken breasts into flour and spice mixture. In a deep-frying pan, add olive oil. Brown chicken until golden brown. Add garlic. Remove chicken breasts and place each piece into a large roasting dish. Bake chicken at 325 degrees F for about 30 minutes or until the poultry is not pink inside. Drizzle a mixture of orange juice, extra virgin olive oil, and rosemary oil over chicken. Place back in oven for about 5 minutes. Remove from oven and garnish with sprigs of rosemary and orange slices.

Makes 6 servings.

Tuna Noodle Casserole

❖ ❖ ❖

Enter the twentieth-century classic tuna noodle casserole. When I was a kid, my mom made this with egg noodles, canned peas, condensed mushroom soup, and canned tuna packed in oil. For a crunch on top it was potato chips. Welcome to the new age tuna noodle casserole. I'm talking healthier fare, including whole grain pasta, organic milk, frozen peas, seasoned bread crumbs, real butter, fresh herbs, and essential oils for a kick of earthy zest.

2 cups organic half-and-half
1 tablespoon all-purpose flour
¼ cup Parmesan or all-natural Cheddar cheese, shredded
2 cups cooked whole grain rotini, drained
1 cup green peas, frozen, thawed
1–2 (3.5-ounce) cans albacore tuna, water-packed, drained (I used one can; you can substitute one can of tuna with fresh carrots, broccoli, and mushrooms, chopped for a meatless casserole.)
2 tablespoons fresh Italian herbs
½ cup Parmesan cheese, shredded
1 drop basil essential oil
1 drop lemon essential oil
2 tablespoons extra virgin olive oil
2 tablespoons European-style butter, melted
Ground pepper to taste
Fresh chives and sliced tomatoes for garnish

In a saucepan mix half-and-half, flour, and cheese. Cook until the white sauce comes to a boil. Remove from the stovetop. Pour into a bowl. Add cooked pasta, peas, and tuna. Add herbs. Put into an ungreased 8-inch by 8-inch square baking dish.

Bake at 350 degrees F for about 20 minutes. Remove. Top with mixture of cheese, basil and lemon oils, extra virgin olive oil and drizzle with butter. Add pepper. Bake for several more minutes until golden brown and cheese is melted. Remove from oven. Cool for about 10 minutes. Cuts nicely in squares or you can dish up in ramekins. Sprinkle with chives and tomatoes.

Makes 8 to 10 servings.

This casserole re-do is full of flavors and the texture is oh-so creamy. Paired with a kale and spinach salad and warm whole grain rolls dipped in olive oil is heaven. This new, improved casserole won't cause any food fasts. Savor the comfort of this super fall or winter dish that will make the kid in you (or your children) smile.

AROMATIC DESSERTS

My choice desserts in the twenty-first century often are a twist from the twentieth-century classic sweet comfort foods. My mom baked sweet-smelling cakes, cookies, pies, and puddings from scratch. But my dishes include different ingredients.

These days, I make desserts that are wholesome and bursting with flavor. Thanks to essential oils, citrus, floral, mint, and spice varieties, you can get taste and some antioxidants, too. Using citrus rind, edible flowers, mint sprigs, and whole spices are preferred but sometimes I do not have all of these ingredients in my kitchen. That's when essential oils, like lemon, are a blessing.

Double Chocolate Cupcakes with Ginger Frosting
Coconut Geranium Cookies
Orange Crème Brûlée with Chocolate Shavings
Cinnamon Rice Pudding

Double Chocolate Cupcakes
with Ginger Frosting

As a child growing up in the 1960s, I had my share of chocolate cupcakes and honestly, Hostess cupcakes with the creamy white filling, dark chocolate glaze, and white squiggly line on top were my favorite. Once I ended up being a Food Network channel groupie, I morphed into a fussier foodie. Homemade cupcakes infused with citrus oil and coated with a spicy ginger oil frosting impressed a group of friends at my cabin. That event ended my days of buying and eating packaged cupcakes. Chocolate cup-cakes with a ginger oil frosting are a scented indulgence to your nose. Once you get a whiff of the orange note and warm spice, and taste it, like me, there's no turning back.

1½ cups flour
½ cup sugar
¼ cup cocoa
1 teaspoon baking soda
½ teaspoon salt
1 egg
¼ cup olive oil
1 tablespoon vinegar (your choice of type)
½ cup orange juice [I use a toothpick drop of orange
    essential oil]
1 teaspoon vanilla extract
½ teaspoon Irish cream extract
½ cup chocolate chips
1 tablespoon espresso coffee powder
12 to 16 Hershey's Kisses

Preheat oven to 375 degrees F. Paper line muffin cups. In a mixing bowl, combine flour, sugar, cocoa, and baking soda. Make a well in the center. Stir in egg, olive oil, vinegar, orange juice, and flavorings. Blend. Add chocolate chips and coffee powder. Pour batter into prepared muffin cups until each is half full. Place one Hershey's in the center of each batter in cup. Spoon remaining batter evenly on top of each kiss to cover. Bake 18 minutes or until cake springs back when lightly touched, cool.

Makes 12 to 16.

(Courtesy: *Baking Sensational Sweets with California Olive Oil*, by Gemma Sanita Sciabica)

GINGER FROSTING

1 cup confectioners sugar, sifted
2 tablespoons low-fat organic milk or half-and-half
1 teaspoon honey
1 drop ginger essential oil
½ cup crystallized ginger, chopped

Combine sugar, milk, and honey. Add ginger oil. Blend using a mixer or by hand until smooth and creamy. Use a pastry piper and frost each cupcake. Top with small bits of crystallized ginger.

Coconut Geranium Cookies

One Saint Patrick's Day, I took a leap of faith and drove over the mountain to attend a book signing. The road was icy, cars were moving at a snail's pace, and a couple of times I mumbled, "I'm turning back."

Once at the bookstore I was greeted with a display of cookie bits and iced berry tea in mini paper cups. I was not chill. My fantasy was to serve fresh cinnamon scones with a pot of hot tea and mugs. Well, that's the way the cookie crumbles. Here's a chewy decadent coconut cookie with a floral essential oil icing recipe inspired by the bittersweet bookstore escapade.

5 tablespoons all-purpose flour (King Arthur's Flour)
1/4 cup granulated white sugar
6 ounces sweetened condensed milk (Carnation)
1 capful pure vanilla extract
7–8 ounces (approximately 2½ cups) sweetened
*   coconut, premium (Baker's)*
2 egg whites
2 tablespoons lemon rind

ICING

8 ounces confectioners sugar (use more if you like a
*   thicker consistency)*
1 drop geranium essential oil
1 teaspoon maple syrup or honey
1 drop pure vanilla extract

For cookies: In a large bowl, combine flour, sugar, milk, and extract. Fold in coconut. Set aside. In a mixing bowl, beat egg whites until stiff. Fold in coconut mixture. Add lemon rind. Use ⅓-cup size cookie scooper to make the cookies alike and place cookie dough on a cookie sheet (parchment paper is nice to avoid sticking).

Bake at 325 degrees F for approximately 15–20 minutes or until bottoms are golden and cookies are firm. Remove immediately Dust cookies with confectioners sugar.

Makes about 10 to 12 cookies, depending on the size you choose.

For Icing: To add an elegant, flavorful touch, make icing (recipe ingredients above). In a bowl combine sugar, oil, maple syrup or honey, and extract until smooth. Drizzle on top of cookies or dip bottoms of cookies in the icing. Let firm. Store in a container.

Orange Crème Brûlée with Chocolate Shavings

Crème brûlée, a rich custard with a crunchy, burnt sugar topping, is a popular and sophisticated dessert. This decadent delight has roots that go back centuries to European cuisine. Back in the 1980s, this light, creamy custard was in demand in French restaurants. And several years ago, this dessert was a pipe dream in my kitchen because I didn't have the chef confidence to create an eye-opening brûlée, which calls for using a torch or broiler turned on high. But I changed.

One summer, a fun-loving neighbor invited me, and my dog, over for a barbecue dinner. I brought a store-bought custard pie, the kind in the frozen food aisle that you bake. Slices of pie topped with whipped cream (yes, the kind in the can) were doable, but I knew I should have tried to make the homemade brûlée and torched the top. That fall I mastered the art of making custard. The custard is best in round or oval-shaped ramekins. To make the sugar topping, you can use a broiler or butane torch—and I chose the first, since it is the safest method if you maintain a keen eye and stay mindful of the task. Topped with a dollop of orange whipped cream, the dessert is heavenly.

2 cups organic half-and-half (premium brand)
½ cup organic low-fat milk
⅓ cup granulated white sugar
4 organic brown eggs, yolks only
1 capful pure vanilla extract (or use vanilla bean from the pod)
2 teaspoons orange rind
Nutmeg (to taste)
¼ cup light brown sugar, ground fine (a bit more if preferred)

TOPPING

Real whipped cream (whip cream until fluffy with peaks)
1 teaspoon maple syrup
1 drop orange essential oil
Dark chocolate shavings (for garnish)

In a saucepan heat half-and-half and milk on medium heat but do not bring to a boil. Set aside. In a bowl, mix white sugar and egg yolks. Pour in milk, slowly, until mixed well. Add vanilla and rind. Pour into 4-ounce ramekins. Sprinkle each with nutmeg. In a pan of cold water place ramekins. Bake at 350 degrees F for about 1 hour or until firm (use a knife to test and when the custard comes out clean on the knife and doesn't jiggle, it is done). Remove ramekins from oven and cool. Place in refrigerator for a few hours. Before serving, whip cream until it's creamy and forms a peak. Add 1 drop of syrup with orange essential oil to 2 cups of whipped cream.

When ready to serve custard, remove ramekins from the refrigerator. Sprinkle tops with brown sugar and place in a 500-degree F oven. Place in a shallow pan with cold water (again), place under broiler. Watch carefully and make sure your ramekins are broiler-safe. In about 1 minute or 2 the sugar will be caramelized. Remove. Place a dollop of orange whipped cream on top. Sprinkle with chocolate shavings.

Serves 4.

Cinnamon Rice Pudding

Rice pudding goes back to the Tudor period in England. A basic rice pudding is made with white rice, whole milk, white sugar, eggs, and vanilla flavoring. It can be cooked in a saucepan on the stovetop or baked in the oven. I was a kid when I first made rice pudding. On a foggy morning in San Jose, I skipped school so I could play chef and cuddle with my new fluffy Norwegian elkhound puppy. I used my mom's recipe. Sitting on the kitchen floor, reading the cookbooks perplexed me. A lot of the recipes were complicated. I didn't understand cooking methods. Decades later, I transformed this Mediterranean dessert with different foods and essential oils. And a furry Australian shepherd kept me company while I changed it up but maintained the memorable cinnamon and vanilla aroma and flavor with a twist of lemon oil for a tart bite.

1 cup brown rice, cooked
2½ cups organic half-and-half
2 large brown eggs, beaten
¼ cup sugar, pure cane granulated white
1 teaspoon vanilla extract
1 drop cinnamon essential oil
1 cup dried cranberries
½ cup walnuts, chopped

TOPPING

2 cups real whipped cream
1 drop lemon essential oil
1 tablespoon maple syrup or honey

Mix cooked rice and half-and-half in a bowl. Add eggs and sugar. Stir well. Add vanilla and cinnamon oil. Fold in dried fruit. Pour into ramekins. Place in 8-inch by 8-inch dish filled with cold water. Bake pudding at 325 degrees F for about 1 hour and 15 minutes or until set. Cool and top with nuts. Top with a dollop of whipped cream mixed well with maple syrup and a tiny drip of lemon oil. Good served warm or cold.

Serves 4.

FINAL ESSENTIAL OILS NOTES

Essential oil use is blossoming—whether it be for its therapeutic uses or in cooking and baking. The key to essential oils is awareness. As long as you only buy pure essential oils from a source you trust, you'll soon join the legions of people who have adopted the oils into their daily lives, from post-hippie boomers to adventure-seeking millennials—and everyone else in between. It's called bonding with Mother Nature's goodness for the body, mind, and spirit. And remember, your nose knows best.

MY MEDITERRANEAN SCENTED GARDEN

Sadly, I missed two booked tours of experiencing the Butchart Gardens in Victoria, British Columbia. So I created my very own Mediterranean aromatic garden. In the summertime I made a sanctuary to provide a scented paradise to calm me during tourist season. Since plants, flowers, and shrubs do not survive long in a cold, dry mountain climate, I took an alternative route with the help of essential oils and aromatherapy.

I covered the deck railing with faux ivy (it lasts year-round) and misted it with orange essential oil to keep the wasps away. Then, I put bunches of artificial lavender spritzed with lavender oil and water into clay pots on the deck. I arranged dozens of river rocks, all sizes, in the back and front yards, and arranged red rock stones for a walking path. Two umbrellas with solar lights were set up with wrought iron tables and chairs. I sprayed bunches of dried eucalyptus with the essential oil and put them in copper pots. I also added a portable essential oil diffuser and used peppermint oil to keep bugs at bay. And solar lights were placed in both front and back looking like an exciting botanical airport runway.

My man-made scented garden in the Sierras was an oasis, where sidewalks and botanical gardens are not plentiful due to our dry climate and short summers. The faux plant–scented flower garden was my sanctuary. Not only did I have sweet solitude, the fragrance took me to a place I love, nourishing the senses, with credit due to the wide world of essential oils. No, it is not a lavender farm, but it is a botanical garden that my nose knows and loves.

ESSENTIAL OILS
RESOURCES

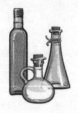

Where Can You Buy Essential Oils

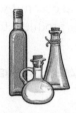

*At early dawn the leaves, of trees are found
bedewed with honey . . . It is always of the best
quality when it is stored in the best flowers.*
—PLINY THE ELDER

As essential oils become more popular for mainstream America and around the globe, people like you and me are willing to go the extra mile to find their favorites to use for health and well-being, in beauty, the household, and cooking and baking.

Some of these essential oil companies carry essential oils, blends, carrier oils, aromatic jewelry, diffusers, beauty items, and more. Also, you can find a wide variety of essential oils and accessories at main on-line stores, such as amazon.com and Walmart.com and other super-stores.

This Resource List can get you started. Make a connection with your go-to source and your quest will be over because that trustworthy find is all you need. I've listed top brands for you, but enjoy your own journey to find your essential oils and aromatherapy soul mate.

ESSENTIAL OIL BEAUTY PRODUCTS

Cali Cosmetics, Inc.
5030 Champion Blvd.
Suite G11192
Boca Raton, FL 33496
www.calicosmetics.com

Candles are made with soy and coconut wax with 15 percent essential oils. Plenty of body and bath products for the aromatherapy experience.

ESSENTIAL OIL AND CARRIER OIL BRANDS

Aura Cacia
c/o Frontier Co-op
P.O. Box 299
3021 78th Street
Norway, IA 52318
www.auracacia.com

Established in 1971. Offers essential oils, single essential oils, blends, body and facial care, diffusers and mists, and accessories.

Eden Garden Essential Oils
1322 Calle Avanzado
San Clemente, CA 92673

Established in 2009, this company offers a variety of products, including room sprays, diffusers, synergy blends, single oils, body care, candles, and more.

doTerra International
389 South 1300 West
Pleasant Grove, UT 84062
www.doterra.com/us/en

Provides high-quality certified pure therapeutic-grade products. Single essential oils, personal care, distillers, accessories, and more.

Kobashi Ltd.
www.kobashi.co.uk

Kobashi Precious Plant Oils, established in 1985. Provides essential oils, carrier oils, and everything you want in oils and scents. Kobashi is a family-run business based on a small farm in the beautiful country-side of Devon. They grow and supply pure authentic essential oils and aromatherapy products.

LorAnn Oils
4518 Aurelius Road
Lansing MI 48910
www.lorannoils.com

Mountain Rose HERBS
P.O. Box 50220
Eugene, OR 97405
www.mountainroseherbs.com

Founded in 1987. USDA-certified single essential oils and blends, aromatic sprays, natural perfumes, natural candles, herbal incense, diffusers, and burners.

NOW Health Food Group, Inc.
www.nowfoods.com

Founded in 1968. They make and distribute natural foods, essential oils, accessories, and more.

Plant Therapy
510 2nd Avenue S
Twin Falls, ID 83301
www.plantherapy.com

A wide selection of essential oils, roll-on blends, carrier oils, KidSafe products, aromatic jewelry, and more.

Young Living
Thanksgiving Point Business Park
3125 Executive Parkway
Lehi, UT 84043
www.youngliving.com

Established in 1993. High-quality essential oils. Many oils distilled in the United States. Essential oils, singles, blends, roll-ons, vitality TMDietary, brands including KidScents, Holiday & Seasonal, and more.

SPECIALTY FOODS

King Arthur Flour
Bakery, Café, Store & School
135 US Rt. 5 South
Norwich, VT 05055
www.kingarthurflour.com/shop

Specialty items for cooking and baking needs, including flavorings, a variety of oils (lemon, orange), extracts, and more.

Nick Sciabica & Sons
2150 Yosemite Blvd.
Modesto, CA 95354
www.sunshineinabottle.com

Sciabica specializes in cold-pressed olive oils using varieties of California olives.

AROMATHERAPY ORGANIZATIONS

National Association for Holistic Aromatherapy
6000 S. 5th Avenue
Pocatello, ID 83204
www.naha.org

The NAHA is an educational, nonprofit organization dedicated to enhancing public awareness of the benefits of aromatherapy.

Pacific Institute of Aromatherapy
602 Freitas Pkwy.
San Rafael, CA 94903
www.pacificinstituteofaromatherapy.com

Pacific Institute of Aromatherapy and Original Swiss Aromatics were founded by Dr. Kurt Schnaubelt in 1983. The OSA is one of the pioneer aromatherapy companies in the United States. Provides courses and products.

NATIONAL HEALTH ORGANIZATIONS

American Cancer Society
www.cancer.org

American Heart Association
www.heart.org

NATIONAL FOOD ORGANIZATIONS

National Honey Board
P.O. Box 2189
Longmont, CO 80502
www.honey.com

The National Honey Board was founded in 1987 to enlighten the public about all things honey related, including some recipes with essential oils combined with honey.

North American Olive Oil Association
3301 Route 66, Suite 205, Bldg. C
Neptune, NJ 07753
www.naooa.org

This association is committed to supplying North American consumers with quality products in a fair and competitive environment; providing some recipes with essential oils combined with olive oil.

HEALTH SPAS

Cal-a-Vie Health Spa
29402 Spa Havens Way
Vista, CA 92084
www.cal-a-vie.com

A luxury resort spa. Carries Cal-a-Vie Vinotherapie body care products and Body Bliss essential oils.

Essential oil companies are gaining momentum with mainstream consumers around the world. Since healing oils and aromatherapy are used in a variety of ways, this market is expanding. If you cannot find the essential oil or aromatherapy device you're looking for, most likely it can be found through online shopping at major outlets including amazon.com, Walmart. com and other large stores.

An understanding of how to incorporate culinary essential oils in their stock is a newer and growing phenomenon, whereas, essential oils for external healing purposes have been promoted for years and are therefore more readily available.

There are other essential oil companies that I could have added to this book, but I've provided the pioneers. Also, I've learned companies can and do change, whether by merging or going AWOL. So if any of the companies ghost you, just move on to a similar one and you should find what you need easily. I'm providing a list that works for me and will get you on the essential track. And then you're on your own, ready to go out into the brave old and new world of essential oils, equipped with the knowledge I have shared with you.

Glossary

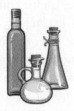

Absolute. Most concentrated form of an essential oil, such as rose and vanilla.

Adulteration. Companies combine pure essentials with a base oil—cutting the integrity of the essential oil—and then sell it impure to make more money. This is done in the olive oil industry.

Aldehydes. A medicinal compound in essential oils, like cinnamon, that lessens inflammation and fights bacteria.

Antibacterial. Inhibits bacteria and germs.

Antidepressant. Helps to lessen depression and boosts emotions and mood.

Antifungal. Gets rid of fungus on the body.

Anti-inflammatory. Lessens inflammation, which is linked to most health ailments and diseases.

Antimicrobial. Prevents microorganisms to grow.

Antioxidant. Slows down oxidation, which can cause premature aging, health ailments, and diseases.

Antiseptic. Fights microbes and halts their growth.

Antispasmodic. Eases spasms and cramps.

Antiviral. Protects against viruses.

Aphrodisiac. Revs up sex drive.

Aromatherapy. Medicinal and therapeutic uses of essential oils through a variety of methods, including inhaling, topically, and ingesting.

Carrier oil. A vegetable oil, such as almond, grape seed, jojoba, and olive oil to dilute essential oils that should not be used undiluted.

Chemotype. Same plant compounds in essential oils, but its component composition is a bit different in some varieties, whereas, a chemist can note the differences.

CO_2 extraction. An herb extraction method using carbon dioxide heat compressed to a critical point, similar to oils made through distillation. Produces higher quality oils not affected by heat.

Cold pressed. A method of extracting essential oils without heat. Examples are citrus oils like lemon and orange.

Decongestant. Gets rid of mucus which causes congestion.

Deodorant. Lessens foul body smell from sweat or lack of bathing.

Diffuser. A device to release aroma molecules from essential oils into the air.

Disinfectant. An aid to fight contamination of germs.

Distillation. A method of extraction of essential oils that uses steam.

Diuretic. Helps get rid of water in the body.

Esters. A medicinal compound in essential oils, like geranium, lavender, and Roman chamomile, that may relax muscles and fight fungal infections.

Extraction. A method by which essential oils are taken from plants whether by distillation, expression, or solvent extraction.

Flavonoids. Antioxidants that belong to the phytochemical family. They are substances found in essential oils that may lower risk of developing cancer, heart disease, and stall aging.

Fomites. Germs on surfaces, which can be contagious.

Food grade. Safe for consumption in food as determined by the Food and Drug Administration.

Hydrocarbons (sesquiterpenes and terpenes). A primary compound in essential oils, such as German chamomile, ginger, lemon, orange, patchouli, and sandalwood, that may guard against bacteria and inflammation.

Hydrosol. Floral water.

Microbes. Germs in water and the environment that can be contagious.

Milliliter. Abbreviated as mL or ml. A liquid measurement in the metric system. Depending on the thickness of the oil, the amount can range from 20 to 25 drops.

Neat. Using a drop of essential oil liquid, undiluted.

Nervine. Helps calm nerves, including anxiety and stress.

Olfactory. Sense of smell.

Phenols. A common potent compound in essential oils, such as basil, that can fight bacteria.

Pipette. A narrow tube attached to a bulb to assist in measuring amounts of liquid, like essential oils.

Roller Balls. A glass tube with a roller on top. It's a convenient device to apply essential oil directly onto the skin.

Skin patch test. A process used to determine whether or not you and an essential oil are compatible. Apply one drop with one-fourth teaspoon carrier oil and put on forearm. After twenty-four hours if there aren't any adverse effects it is safe for use.

Stimulant. Increases circulation in the body.

Synergy. Compounds combined to work together for better results.

Tincture. Herbal material mixed in an alcohol base and used for therapeutic benefits.

Unadulterated. No fake ingredients or substances in an essential oil or absolute. Adulterated oils and absolutes can keep the cost down for the producer but lose their essence for the consumer.

Acknowledgments

A heartfelt thanks goes to essential oil companies, big and small. I am inspired by the forward-thinking people behind the scenes of essential oils and aromatherapy in the United States and around the world. These folks helped me understand how this industry is essential to our total health and well-being today, as it was in ancient times.

As always, I cannot ignore the open-minded aromatherapists, naturopaths, medical doctors, and researchers who understand plant therapy from essential oils and aromatherapy, an ancient medicine that is still used for healing the mind, body, and spirit. When scientific studies and anecdotal evidence show time after time that essential oils are nature's medicine, it's time to wake up and smell the unforgettable scents on this planet!

A special feeling of gratitude goes to organizations, including the National Association for Holistic Aromatherapy, Pacific Institute for Aromatherapy, and all the people behind plant therapy (you know who you are), essential oil gurus who extended a warm and gracious welcome to me—just a health-conscious author-journalist traveling on a road to learn about the land of essential oils and aromatherapy. As I explored the world of plants and its medicinal oils, I always felt at home wherever I was in the world of research. As I wrote this book, much like putting a puzzle together, the pieces began to fit and at the end I saw a whole picture. I learned everything I wanted to know without getting lost in "scientif-ese" or stuck in an advanced chemistry class. I ended up with a nice-size book, not too heavy to carry or needing a dictionary to decode every foreign term.

A profound thanks goes to the Kensington Publishing team, who are behind the core of each book in the *Healing Powers* series. And for this one in particular I am grateful to have gone out of my comfort zone and freshened up the series—for both the reader and me! I am happy to write this book collection that feels like a growing family tree to me. I owe this guide on essential oils to the first book, *The Healing Powers of Vinegar*, which spawned other books to complement it.

And lastly, a big thanks and hug to the followers of the *Healing Powers* series and new readers who are interested in the world of essential oils and want to know which ones to use, for what, and how to use them—without all the technical bells and whistles. I dish up just the facts and fun stuff. I decoded nature's plant therapy pharmacy for me, and you—with a little help from everyone I contacted. Thank you so much.

Notes

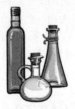

CHAPTER 1:
POWERFUL HEALING OF PLANTS

1. Valerie Ann Worwood, *The Complete Book of Essential Oils and Aromatherapy: Over 800 Natural, Nontoxic, and Fragrant Recipes to Create Health, Beauty and Safe Home and Work Environments* (Novato, CA: New World Library, 1991), 1.
2. Kathie Keville, *Aromatherapy for Dummies* (Hoboken, NJ: Wiley, 1999), 16.
3. David Stewart, Ph.D., *Healing Oils of the Bible* (Marble Hill, MO: Care Publications, 2003), 30.
4. Ali Baber et al., "Essential Oils Used in Aromatherapy: A Systematic Review." *Asian Pac J Trop Biomed*, 5 (8) (August 2015): 601–611. DOI: org/10:1016/apjtb. 2015.05.007.

CHAPTER 2:
HISTORY OF ESSENTIAL OILS

1. Stewart, *Healing Oils of the Bible*, 97.
2. Ibid., 101–108.
3. Ibid., 96.
4. Cal Orey, *The Healing Powers of Vinegar* (New York: Kensington, 2000), 13.

Chapter 3:
Basil

1. Keville, *Aromatherapy for Dummies*, 290–291.
2. Rajesh K. Joshi et al., "Chemical Composition and Antimicrobial Activity of the Essential Oil of Ocimum L. (sweet basil) from Western Ghats of North West Karmataka, India." *Anc Sci Life*, 33 (3) (Jan–Mar 2014): 151–156. DOI: 10.4103/0257-7941.144618.

Chapter 4:
Cedarwood

1. Stewart, *Healing Oils of the Bible*, 288.
2. Antoine Saab et al., "Phytochemical Analysis and Cytotoxicity Toward Multi-Drug-Resistant Leukemia Cells of Essential Oils Derived from Labanes Medicinal Plants." *Planta Med*, 18 (Dec 2012): 927–931. DOI: 1055/s 0032-1327896. Epub 2012. Nov. 14.

Chapter 5:
Chamomile

1. K. Janmejai et al., "Chamomile: A Herbal Medicine of the Past with Bright Future." *Mol Med Report*, 3 (6) (Nov 1, 2010): 895-901. DOI: 10:3892/mmr.2010.377.

Chapter 6:
Cinnamon

1. A. Khan et al., "Cinnamon Improves Glucose and Lipid of People with Type 2 Diabetes." *Diabetes Care*, 12 (Dec 26, 2003): 3215–3218).

Chapter 7:
Eucalyptus

1. M. H. Salari et al., "Antibacterial Effects of Eucalyptus Globus Leaf Extract on Pathogenic Bacteria Isolated from Specimens with

Respiratory Tract Disease." *Clin Microbiol and Infec*, 12 (2) (2006): 194–196.

CHAPTER 9:
GINGER

1. Keville, *Aromatherapy for Dummies*, 154.
2. Arshad H. Rahmani et al., "Active Ingredients of Ginger as Potent Candidates in the Prevention and Treatment of Disease Via Modulation of Biological Activities." *Int J Physiol Pathophysiol Pharmacol*, 6 (2) (2014): 125–136.

CHAPTER 10:
JASMINE

1. Olga Sergeeva et al., "Fragrant Dioxane Derivatives Identify1 Subunit-Containing GABA Receptors." *J Biol Chem*, 285 (31) (July 30, 2010): 23985–23993.
2. Tapanee Hongratanawor akit et al., "Stimulating Effect of Aromatherapy Massage with Jasmine Oil." *Nat Prod Commun*, 5 (1) (Jan 2010): 157–162.

CHAPTER 11:
LAVENDER

1. Robert Shellie et al., "Characterization of Lavender Essential Oils by Using Gas Chromatography—Mass Spectrometry with Correlation in Linear Retention Indices and Comparison with Comprehensive Two-Dimensional Gas Chromatography." *Journal of Chromatography*, 970 (1–2) (Sept 12, 2002): 2251.
2. S. Kasper et al., "An Orally Administered Lavandula Oil Preparation (Silexan) for Anxiety Disorder and Related Conditions: An Evidence Based Review." *Int J Psychiatry Clin Pract*, 17, Suppl. 1 (Nov 2013): 15–22. DOI: 0.3109/13651501.2013.813555.

Chapter 12:
Lemon

1. Handan Dalia, "Chemical Composition of the Essential Oils of Variegated Pink-fleshed Lemon (Citrus x limon L. Burm. F.) and Their Anti-inflammatory and Antimicrobial Activities." *Zeitsbrift fur Naturforschung C: J Biosci*, 68 (7–8) (Jan 2013): 275–284.

Chapter 13:
Orange

1. Hang Xiao et al., "Monodemethylated polymethoxflavones from Sweet Orange (Citrus sinensis) Peel Inhibit Growth of Human Lung Cancer Cells by Apoptosis." *Mol Nut Food Res*, 53 (3) (Mar 2009): 398–406. DOI: 10:1002/mnfr.200800057.
2. Kang-Ming Chang et al., "Aromatherapy Benefits Autonomic Nervous System Regulation for Elementary School Facility in Taiwan." *Evid Based Complement Alternat Med* (2011): 946357.
3. Jimbo Daiki et al., "Effect of Aromatherapy on Patients with Alzheimer's Disease." *Psychogeriatrics* (4) (Dec 9, 2009): 173–179. DOI: 10.1111/j. 1479-8301/2009.0099.x.

Chapter 15:
Peppermint

1. Briggs P. Hawryflack et al., "Inhaled Peppermint Oil for Postop Nausea in Patients Undergoing Cardia Surgery." *Nursing*, 46 (7) (July 2016): 61–67. DOI: 10971oi. NURSE 882.38607.5u.
2. Worwood, *The Complete Book of Essential Oils*, 459.

Chapter 16:
Rose

1. Stewart, *Healing Oils of the Bible*, 127.
2. Forzaneh Barati et al., "The Effect on Anxiety in High Risk Patents." *Nephrourol Mon*, 8 (5) (Sept 2016): e38347.

CHAPTER 19:
SANDALWOOD

1. Keville, *Aromatherapy for Dummies*, 156.

CHAPTER 20:
SPEARMINT

1. Abdullah I. Husssain et al., "Chemical Composition, and Antioxidant and Antimicrobial Activities of Essential Oil of Spearmint (Mentha spicata L.) From Pakistan." *Journal of Essential Oil Research*, 22 (1) (2010): 78–84. DOI: 10.1080/10412905.2010.9700269.
2. Ecancermedical science (2013): 7290. DOI: 10.3332/cancer/ 2013. 290. Epub.2013 published online January 31.

CHAPTER 21:
TEA TREE

1. C. F. Carson, K. A. Hammer, et al., "Melaleuca Alternifolic (Tea Tree) Oil: A Review Antimicrobial and Other Medicinal Properties." *Clin Microbiol Rev*, 19 (1) (Jan 2006): 50–62. DOI: 10:11281 CMR.19.1.40-62.2006.

CHAPTER 22:
VANILLA

1. B. F. Shyamala, K. Anuradhak et al., "Vanilla—Its Science Cultivation, Curing, Chemistry, and Nutraceutical Properties." *Crit Rev Food Sci Nutr*, 53 (12) (2013): 1250–1276. DOI: 10.1080/10408396. 2011 563879.
2. B. F. Shyamala et al., "Studies on Antioxidant Activities of Natural Vanilla Extract and Its Constituent Compounds through in vitro Models." *J Agri Food Chem*, 55 (19) (Oct 2007): 7738–7743. DOI: 10. 1021/jf071349+.
3. Ashan Sho et al., "Evaluation of Antidepressant Activity of Vanillin in Mice." *Indian J Pharmacol*, 45 (2) (Mar–Apr 2013): 141–144. DOI: 10.4103/1253-7613:108292.

CHAPTER 23:
AROMATIC AGE-FIGHTING OILS

1. National Cancer Institute, "Aromatherapy with Essential Oils (PDQ®)—Health Professional Version." Accessed September 31, 2018.
2. Moss M. Cook et al., "Aromas of Rosemary and Lavender Essential Oils Differentially Affect Cognition and Mood in Healthy Adults." *Int J Neurosci*, 113 (1) (Jan 2003): 15–38.

CHAPTER 24:
THE SLIMMING ESSENTIALS

1. A. R. Hirsh et al., "Weight Reduction Through Inhalation of Odorants." *J Neurol Orthop Med Surg*, 16 (1995): 28–31.
2. Hiroki Harada et al., "Linalool Odor-Induced Anxiolytic Effects in Mice." *Front Behav Neurosci*, published online. Accessed October 23, 2018. DOI: 10.3389/fnbeh. 2018 00241.

CHAPTER 25:
HOME CURES FROM YOUR KITCHEN

1. The editors of FC&A Medical Publishing, *The Folk Remedy Encyclopedia: Olive Oil, Vinegar, Honey and 1001 Other Home Remedies* (Peachtree City, GA: Frank W. Cawood and Associates, Inc. 2004), 368.
2. A. C. Ford, N. J. Talley, et al., "Effect of Fibre, Antispasmodics, and Peppermint Oil in the Treatment of Irritable Bowel Syndrome: Systematic Review and Met-Analysis." *BMJ*, 337 (2008): 2313. DOI: 10.1136/bmj.
3. Andrea St. Cyr et al., "Efficacy and Tolerability of STOPAIN for a Migraine Attack." *Frontiers Neruol*, 201 (5) (Feb 4, 2015): 11. Published online. DOI: 10. 3389/fneur. 2015.00011.

4. Reneau Z. Peurifoy, *Updated and Revised Anxiety, Phobias & Panic: A Step-by-Step Program for Regaining Control of Your Life* (New York: Warner Books, 1998), 145.

CHAPTER 28
THE JOY OF COOKING WITH EDIBLE OILS

1. FDA U.S. Food & Drug Administration. accessdata.fda.gov/scripts/cdrh/cfdocs/cfcfr/CFRSearch.cfm?fr=182.20

Selected Bibliography

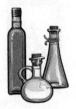

Keville, Kathie. *Aromatherapy for Dummies.* Hoboken, NJ: Wiley, 1999.

Peurifoy, Reneau Z. *Updated and Revised Anxiety, Phobias, & Panic: A Step-by-Step Program for Regaining Control of Your Life.* New York: Warner, 2005.

Sanita Sciabica, Gemma. *Cooking with California Olive Oil: Treasured Family Recipes.* Modesto, CA: Gemma Sanita Sciabica, 1998.

———. *Baking with California Olive Oil: Dolci and Biscotti Recipes.* Modesto, CA: Gemma Sanita Sciabica, 2002.

———. *Cooking with California Olive Oil: Recipes from the Heart for the Heart.* Modesto, CA: Gemma Sanita Sciabica, 2009.

Schnaubelt, Kurt. *The Healing Intelligence of Essential Oils: The Science of Advanced Aromatherapy.* Rochester, VT: Healing Arts Press, 2011.

Worwood, Valerie Ann. *The Complete Book of Essential Oils and Aromatherapy: Over 800 Natural, Nontoxic, and Fragrant Recipes to Create Health, Beauty, and Safe Home and Work Environments.* Novato, CA: New World Library, 1991.

Zielinskin, Eric. *The Healing Powers of Essential Oils: Soothe Inflammation, Boost Mood, Prevent Autoimmunity, and Feel Great in Every Way.* New York: Harmony, 2018.

Connect with U s

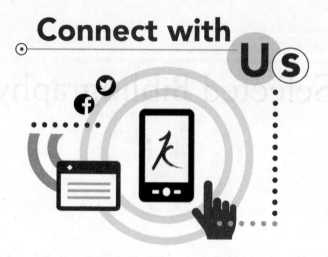

Visit us online at
KensingtonBooks.com
to read more from your favorite authors, see books
by series, view reading group guides, and more.

Join us on social media

for sneak peeks, chances to win books and prize packs,
and to share your thoughts with other readers.

facebook.com/kensingtonpublishing
twitter.com/kensingtonbooks

Tell us what you think!

To share your thoughts, submit a review,
or sign up for our eNewsletters, please visit:
KensingtonBooks.com/TellUs.